How to Care for Your Back

HOW TO CARE FOR YOUR BACK

Hugo A. Keim, M.D.

Prentice-Hall, Inc., Englewood Cliffs, New Jersey 07632

ISBN 0-13-403162-8 {A REWARD BOOK : PBK.}

Grateful acknowledgment is made to CIBA Pharmaceutical
Company for permission to reprint art. © Copyright
1980 CIBA Pharmaceutical Company, Division of
CIBA-GEIGY Corporation. Reprinted with permission
from CLINICAL SYMPOSIA by Hugo A. Keim, M.D., and
W. H. Kirkaldy-Willis, M.D., illustrated by Frank
H. Netter, M.D. All rights reserved.

Printed in the United States of America
Prentice-Hall International, Inc., London
Prentice-Hall of Australia, Pty. Ltd., Sydney
Prentice-Hall of Canada, Ltd., Toronto
Prentice-Hall of India Private Ltd., New Delhi
Prentice-Hall of Japan, Inc., Tokyo
Prentice-Hall of Southeast Asia Pte. Ltd., Singapore
Whitehall Books Limited, Wellington, New Zealand

Library of Congress Cataloging in Publication Data
Keim, Hugo A.
    How to care for your back.
    Includes index.
    1. Backache. 2. Back—Care and hygiene. I. Title.
RD768.K4   617'.56   81-8498
ISBN 0-13-403170-9   AACR2

To my parents, family, and loving friends, who have so strongly supported me through both good times and bad.

Contents

Preface

This is a no-nonsense book about your back. It is being written because I have spent most of my life learning to understand the problems of the human spine and why we are burdened with such an extremely high incidence of back pain. My curiosity has always been aroused by the incredible anatomy of the human spine and how marvelously our bodies have been created.

Why do humans have so much difficulty with their backs? Back problems are growing at an alarming and precipitous rate. Backaches are the second largest pain problem in our society, secondary only to headaches. The United States Public Health Service estimates that in 1978, between twelve and fifteen million people experienced impairments and chronic pains in the lower back that resulted in visits to physicians. Visits for back pain rank second only to routine checkups. Back complaints are up an incredible 25 percent from the survey done only eight years earlier. The Public Health Service also says that impairments of the back are the most frequent cause of activity limitation in persons under age forty-five, and rank as the third most common cause of disability, after heart and arthritic conditions, in patients forty-five and over.

Almost everyone, at some time in his or her life, will experience back pain and be incapacitated by it. It is estimated that on any given day over six and a half million people are in bed in the United States because of back pain. Approximately four out of every five people in the U.S. can expect to have back pain sometime in their life, and new cases of back pain appear at the rate of approximately one and a half million per month.

Acknowledgments

I would like to thank several people for their tremendous help and assistance in stimulating me to proceed with this book. First of all, I would like to express my appreciation to my teachers, especially the late Drs. Robert B. McElvenny and John J. Fahey of Northwestern University Medical School, who were the first professors to make me aware of the importance of low back pain in orthopaedics. They kindled my intense interest in this problem. I would also like to thank Dr. Frank E. Stinchfield for his tremendous support and help during my years at the Columbia-Presbyterian Medical Center, and for his interest in helping young people forge ahead in new areas.

My thanks to Mr. Dennis Fawcett, who served as my editor during publication, and also to my typist, Ms. Anne Kerrigan, for her excellent work over numerous revisions and thousands of pages of typing. Ms. Anne Trench has also greatly assisted me in combining proper syntax and style.

Some excellent illustrations by Dr. Frank Netter have been reproduced here with the kind permission of the CIBA Pharmaceutical Company of Summit, New Jersey. They come from a monograph I originally wrote in 1973 and revised in 1980 with Dr. William Kirkaldy-Willis. The booklet is called *Low Back Pain*, and has been used by medical students and educators throughout the world.

Other artwork in this book was provided by Mr. Robert Demarest and Mr. John Karapelou. It is outstanding and proves that one picture is worth a thousand words.

God bless my secretary and close friend, Gloria Curry, for her continued encouragement and moral support. Also, Dr. Alexander Garcia, my Chief at the New York Orthopaedic Hospital for his generous advice and counsel.

Finally, I would like to thank my family and friends, who have put up with exasperating and difficult periods and who understood my need to give birth to this book.

Introduction

Backache is a stranger to no one. It has no regard for age, sex, or social status. Only a victim of backache can really understand the sense of helplessness that occurs when a vigorous adult is struck down and bedridden because of severe back pain. In most cases the ailment is temporary; however, in some cases it becomes so distressing that several weeks a year are spent in bed. Dressing becomes almost torturous, and a visit to the bathroom becomes a major venture. Simple things such as sitting in a chair or trying to sit at a desk can become most agonizing. Even when the pain subsides, people who have previously had backaches always worry that any future movement or activity will suddenly trigger a recurrence.

Besides causing personal aggravation, painful backs are extremely costly. In the United States, over ninety million workdays per year are lost because of back problems. Americans spend over five billion dollars a year for tests and treatment from a confusing array of people who claim to be able to treat their backs, including acupuncturists, osteopaths, chiropractors, neurologists, orthopaedists, and physical therapists, not to mention self-styled bogus healers.

People throughout the world are bothered with back pain. It is most common in the industrialized societies, where daily strenuous work is no longer routine. Interestingly, on South Sea islands, where the natives are still engaged in strenuous physical labor, very few cases of back pain are reported.

I hope this book will help the average person understand spinal problems, how to prevent them before they start, and how to deal with them if they should occur.

The Purpose of This Book

On July 14, 1980, *Time* magazine ran a cover article on back pain. The feature story of seven pages was the result of intensely accurate and detailed research by *Time* editors. In that article, I had the privilege of being quoted several times and of presenting my views. Shortly thereafter, several major publishing houses asked me to write a book that would be directed strictly to the layperson who needed to know something more about back problems. I decided to write this book in the hope that my efforts will help to keep patients *out* of doctors' offices and in good spinal health for their entire lives.

This book is not intended to be read from cover to cover as a novel. It is a reference book, with each chapter outlining a specific problem and how to deal with it. If difficulties arise, you can refer to a chapter for prevention, for treatment, or even for self-diagnosis. A section on how to treat your own back before seeking professional advice is offered and should be of great help to patients.

In addition, a preventive group of five exercises which I have compiled should help you to stay fit and avoid back pain, *if done daily*. I call these the KPEs (Keim *Preventive* Exercises). In addition, if you do experience back pain, for whatever reason, I recommend six remedial exercises, which I call the PREs (Pain-*Relieving* Exercises). I am convinced that a person who does the five KPEs *daily* (which would take about twelve to fifteen minutes) will probably never need to worry about chronic back pain. Most victims of long-standing back pain should obtain marked relief by doing the six PREs *daily!*

Occasionally, however, self-help will not solve the entire problem, and it will be necessary to seek out professional care. To this end, there is a chapter on how to choose your doctor and on what to expect from a routine back examination. In addition, there is a section on various treatment modalities for back pain, whether acute or chronic, and what to expect before you consent to treatment.

American medicine is advancing at an extremely alarming rate. For too many years patients have been intimidated by health-care professionals' knowledge. Often patients are afraid to ask questions for fear of sounding foolish. I hope this book will encourage patients to ask questions and to be more aware of what can happen to them. I hope I can show them what good medical care is and encourage them to demand that care from their doctor. Patients should not be afraid to ask questions or to insist on first-class care. In this modern society, that is the least that can be expected. After all, it is your body, and you should know *How to Care for Your Back!*

**Life is short
and the art long.
The occasion instant,
experiment perilous,
decision difficult.**
Hippocrates

One

PRACTICAL ANATOMY OF THE SPINE

DEFINITION OF TERMS

For many years people talking about back pain have bandied about terms that are confusing and imprecise. For example, the term *lumbago* has been used for centuries to refer to any type of pain that occurs in the lumbar spine, the lowest part of the back. The term is really not diagnostic at all, but merely means pain in the back. *Sciatica* is a much more precise term, but should be used only in reference to *problems that irritate the sciatic nerve*, the longest nerve in the body. The sciatic nerve can be pressed upon from any one of its roots of origin inside the spine, since it is made up of the lowest two lumbar as well as the upper three sacral nerve roots. A great number of different conditions can cause pressure on those nerve roots—leading to sciatica.

Another common term is *disc disease*. Many people talk about slipped discs and herniated discs. Much of this terminology is confusing because the discs, which are shock absorbers located between the vertebrae, really *do not slip!* Lumping most spinal problems together under the term of *slipped disc* is generally confusing and inaccurate.

For years we have heard people talk about pinched nerves in their back. Nerves can become pinched or trapped, causing specific problems in the spine.

People also occasionally talk about their back going out. They are usually referring to an acute muscular strain or even a muscle tear caused by strenuous activity. People's backs really don't "go out," but a specific injury occurs to some area of the back, causing pain.

1

Finally, there is a new term in the medical field, *spinal stenosis*. The word *stenosis* means a narrowing or constriction of any area. We have learned in recent years that a great number of back problems occur with age as a result of narrowing within the spinal canal and direct pressure on the nerve roots. There are dozens of other terms used to refer to back disorders, but the ones mentioned are those most often misunderstood. Others will be defined in the course of this book so that you can use them accurately.

THE NORMAL SPINE

A basic knowledge of the anatomy of the spine is essential in understanding what is normal and what is abnormal. The spinal column consists of blocks (the vertebrae) stacked one on top of the other. There are thirty-three vertebrae in all: seven in the neck region, the cervical spine; twelve in the thoracic region, to which the ribs are attached; and five in the lumbar region, the area just above the pelvis. Below the lumbar region are five sacral vertebrae, which are usually fused into one bone called the sacrum. Finally, there are four coccygeal vertebrae which are often fused into one, but sometimes consist of two, three, or four bones which stay loose.

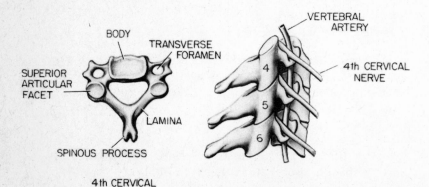

Figure 1–1. Drawing of the vertebrae of the cervical spine (neck). Notice in the side view how the vertebral artery runs through a small hole in the vertebrae and is in close proximity to the cervical nerves as they exit from the spinal cord.

Because the sacrum and coccyx are each considered as single units, humans have essentially twenty-six active vertebrae. These vertebrae are held together by a marvelously exact system of ligaments, fibrous structures that connect bone to bone. These and the interposed cartilages and muscles act with tremendous precision to hold the vertebrae together and keep the spinal column from collapsing.

In the neck the seven cervical vertebrae are generally small. They provide protection for the spinal cord, which is vulnerable in this region (Fig. 1–1).

There are twelve thoracic vertebrae, each of which is joined to a rib (Fig. 1–2). The ribs have multiple functions; they work as a bellows, expanding and contracting with the action of the rib muscles to help us in breathing. Aside from protecting

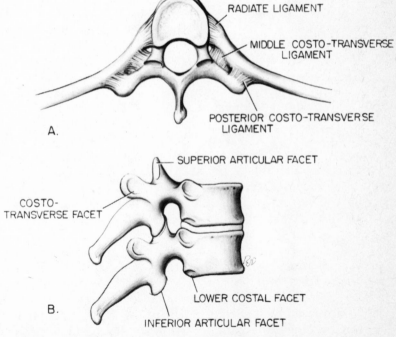

Figure 1–2. Drawing of typical thoracic vertebrae. Notice in the side view how two vertebrae together make up the small foramen or window through which the nerves exit the spine. Notice also the many ligaments which hold the ribs against the body of the vertebrae and against the posterior portion of the vertebrae itself.

the important structures inside our chest (the lungs, heart, and major blood vessels), the ribs protect the spine from injury.

In this book we are going to concentrate on the lumbar area, since the majority of back pain occurs in this region. The lumbar vertebrae are constructed to resist the weight and stress of the torso, which rests above them. Through these vertebrae pass the nerve roots, which give rise to the important nerves running down our legs, especially the femoral and sciatic nerves (Fig. 1–3).

In the embryo, the spinal cord extends all the way down to the sacrum, but by the time the baby is born, it only reaches the level of the third lumbar vertebra. Spinal cord growth does not keep pace with vertebral growth and, as a result, the spinal cord is found at higher levels in the spinal canal with each year, until age twelve, when spinal growth is complete.

Because of this unequal growth, the nerve roots in the lower part of the spinal cord slant downward from the spinal cord at about the level of the first lumbar vertebra and then run down through the spinal canal in the lumbar region, where they exit from between each pair of vertebrae. The nerve roots in this region form the nerves to the lower parts of our body (Fig. 1–4).

Between each pair of lumbar vertebrae there is a small window formed by the lowest (inferior) portion of the arch of the upper vertebrae and the upper portion of the arch from the lower vertebrae (Fig. 1–3). It is through this window or foramen that the spinal nerves pass. Within the foramen, nerves are particularly vulnerable to pressure or damage from conditions such as tumors, fractures, or herniated discs. Conditions that disturb the normal exit of the spinal nerves through these foramina (windows) are called *nerve root entrapment syndromes* and are commonly referred to as pinched nerves.

The facets are small joints made up of a superior articular process from the lower vertebrae and an inferior articular process from the upper vertebrae. There is a facet joint on both the right and left sides of *each pair of vertebrae.* When degenerative changes, such as arthritis, form in these joints, they can become quite painful. Also, they can be congenitally deformed and lie in different planes, which we refer to as *facet tropism* (Fig 1–3). Tropisms can cause abnormal motions and faulty mechanics of the spine, leading to back pain.

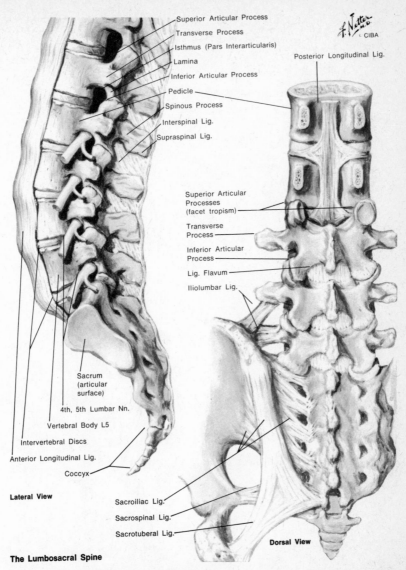

Figure 1–3. The lumbar spine showing in the side view the nerves coming from the lower lumbar vertebrae. In addition, notice the intervertebral disc between each pair of vertebral bodies, and also the ligaments holding the vertebrae together. On the dorsal view, notice how the facet joints can vary in different planes (facet tropism). (Copyright © 1980 CIBA Pharmaceutical Company

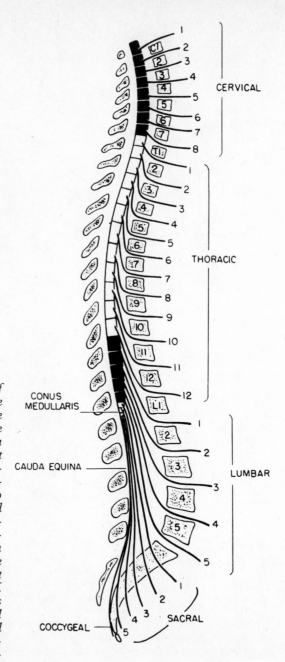

Figure 1–4. Diagram of the exit of the nerve roots from the entire spinal cord. Notice how the nerves exit in the cervical spine at right angles to the spinal cord. In the thoracic spine they start to slant downward slightly, and in the lumbar spine and the sacrum, they slant down a long distance before they make their exit from the spine itself. The reason for this is the ascent of the spinal cord during rapid growth in early fetal development and childhood.

Between each pair of vertebrae is a major joint that has a cartilaginous disc. This disc separates the two vertebrae and acts as a shock absorber. Each disc consists of an outer fibrous portion called the anulus fibrosus, and an inner, puttylike section called the nucleus pulposus. This central section of the disc often leaks out through the rear portion of the anulus, to cause what is commonly known as a slipped disc. The disc has not really slipped but leaked, causing a hernia formed by jellylike material that has come from the disc, just like putty comes out of a putty gun.

The disc between each pair of vertebrae helps create a space between vertebral bodies and holds open the little window or intervertebral foramen so that the nerves can pass safely out to the lower limbs and perform their function (Fig. 1–3). If a disc is injured or degenerates, the vertebral bodies above and below that disc will narrow, closing down the window, causing pinching or entrapment of that particular spinal nerve.

THE SPINE IN CHILDHOOD, ADOLESCENCE, AND ADULTHOOD

The average girl born today can expect to live until her mid-eighties and the average boy until his late seventies. Thus, we must learn to protect our bodies so that we do not wear them out in the first forty or fifty years of life.

In childhood the spine is extremely flexible, but by adolescence its elasticity decreases. The ligaments, which hold bone to bone, and the tendons, which hold muscle to bone, become better reinforced and more rigid, holding the spine in proper position. However, during the adult years the material within the spine tends to degenerate, just as rust forms on a car, depending on how much the body is abused.

AGING FACTORS AND OSTEOPOROSIS

Spinal health in old age depends on just how much injury we inflict upon ourselves during our adolescent years when we are generally active athletically, and also on what type of injuries occur to us.

In later adult life, the water content of the intervertebral discs decreases, and the ligaments around the vertebrae become brittle. Another aging factor, especially common in women, is *osteoporosis.* This condition causes a decrease in the mass or weight of the vertebrae, even though they still take up the same amount of space. In most cases osteoporosis is related to aging. It occurs more rapidly in certain individuals than in others, and is possibly of genetic origin.

We have learned a great deal about the effects of exercise and diet through the space program. It seems that when a person is shot off into space, in an area without gravity, osteoporosis increases at an alarming rate. Astronauts must do specific exercises while awake to keep their vertebrae from losing mineral content. NASA studies show that 20 percent of muscle strength is lost after just three days of immobility.

Osteoporosis in Women

There are two specific times in women's lives when muscle weakness and osteoporosis are serious threats—pregnancy and menopause. Some women who have had eight or ten children look old even though they may only be in their early thirties.

Pregnancy is a serious challenge to a woman, but with proper diet and exercise right up to the time of delivery, the birth of a child can be a healthy and pleasant experience.

I see a great number of out-of-shape young mothers who complain of low back pain. They become increasingly swaybacked, which causes pinching of the lumbar nerves as they exit the spine. It is sad to see so many women in their early thirties and forties who are overweight, underexercised, and caught in a vicious cycle of inactivity followed by back pain. *The more their backs hurt, the less active they become. The less active they become, the more their backs hurt!* Sometimes, after three or four pregnancies, their muscle tone is absolutely nil.

The second major threat to a woman occurs during menopause. Menopause, of course, occurs in all women; it is the time when the hormonal cycle slows down. It can begin any time between the ages of forty and fifty. Now that we understand menopause and the biochemical changes that occur, we are more able to counteract its effects with proper food supplements and exercise programs. In Chapter 4 osteoporosis and menopause are discussed in greater detail.

Two

WHY DO WE HAVE BACK PROBLEMS?

In a nutshell, the main reasons for most back problems are emotional stress, improper diet, and lack of exercise. Originally, man walked on all fours, but through some anthropological and evolutionary process, probably over ten million years ago, he began to walk on his hind limbs. Whether the transition was as simple as man standing up to reach for the forbidden fruit in the Garden of Eden, we will never know. However, the fact is that anatomically, we would have been better off had we stayed on all fours!

STRESS

Stress is *the most important single factor causing back pain* in our modern age. The psychologically well-adjusted person who has a normal exercise pattern and does a fair amount of strenuous but well-balanced work, and eats a proper diet, will rarely have serious back problems. However, most of us just don't lead our lives that way! We are usually in a tremendous hurry and under great pressures. We must cope with the stresses of trying to raise a family, providing modern conveniences for our loved ones, and/or competing in the daily work force to try to make a decent living. Too often, we let these pressures build up; they take their toll by surfacing as muscle tension and fatigue. Unfortunately we cannot measure stress as we can measure blood pressure or do a blood cell count. However, we do know that fifty-three million Americans smoke six hundred billion cigarettes per year, and 68 percent of our adult population drinks alcohol. We also know that 100 percent of us experience stress and some of us handle it better than others.

An infant's only concerns are getting fed and being kept warm. Children are exposed to more stressful peer pressure. By age thirty or forty, adults are preoccupied with making a living, social situations, and the burden of raising two or three children. As adults get into their fifties, they "plateau out" and start worrying about losing their jobs, menopause, sexual function, and baldness. They have more bills and taxes to pay, and begin worrying about inflation and its effect on the so-called golden years.

It is well known that excessive stress can lead to drug and alcohol abuse, depression, high blood pressure, overeating and obesity, high cholesterol (leading to heart attacks), and smoking (which causes lung cancer). It can also lead to back pain.

Dr. Hans Selye first coined the term *stress* in 1936 and helped us understand it. When we are under stress, adrenalin causes our bodies to prepare for "fight or flight." While centuries ago we only had to contend with avoiding hungry dinosaurs, we now have family problems, traffic jams, miserable work situations, in-laws, and children that add stresses to our lives, not to mention the stress of living with the threat of nuclear war. It is amazing that most of us cope as well as we do!

Some stressful events exact a greater toll than others. Obviously, the death of a spouse, a divorce, jail term, or loss of a job would be much more stressful than a vacation, Christmas, or a minor traffic violation. It is how you cope with these stresses and how many of them you have to cope with that determines their effect on your health!

About 90 percent of the patients I see with back pain are coping with some major underlying stressful situation that is aggravating their pain. If this situation can be eliminated or improved, the back pain will often improve. That is the reason why most patients with chronic back pain do not do well in their home environment and must be treated in the hospital where they are free of their stressful surroundings.

Coping with stress is a product of both genetics and previous experience. Coping ability can be improved through training and education. I remember the first time I tried to address a large audience—severe stress! Now I do it all the time with a minimum of stress. We can all learn to cope, with experience and by trying to keep cool, as the younger generation constantly advises. With proper training and support—sometimes from professionals—you *can increase your ability to cope* with stress.

DIET

The next important causative factor is improper diet. Although Americans are perhaps the best-fed people in the world today, most of us do not eat nutritionally balanced diets. We eat the foods we like although they may not always be the best foods for us. A great number of Americans are constantly on one type of reducing diet or another. Many of these diets do not provide proper nourishment for our bodies; they are fad diets or consist of pure starvation and deprive us of the vitamins and minerals we need to keep our bodies in good muscular tone.

Our body is a powerhouse, much like any engine. It has to have the proper fuel to function efficiently. If we starve our engine of some of the essential ingredients for proper operation, the engine will fail to work. Because so much of our food is overprocessed, it is often an inadequate source of minerals and vitamins. Thus, people should take some type of vitamin supplements in addition to their regular diet. Even if we do eat well-balanced meals, a vitamin supplement with minerals cannot hurt us and may actually be most helpful. However, it is not true that if one multivitamin is good for you, megadoses must be terrific! Vitamin overdosage can lead to vitamin intoxication and serious problems such as kidney or bladder stones and cataract formation. Although many promote megadoses of vitamin C, the medical community generally considers such dosages to be unsafe. Large doses of any vitamin should never be taken without consulting a doctor first.

EXERCISES

The last and certainly one of the major factors causing back pain is lack of exercise, or as Dr. Hans Kraus puts it, "hypokinesis."

Unfortunately, Americans have learned to become sedentary. Hundreds of years ago, when we lived in a chiefly agricultural society, we were forced to do physical work and thus got daily physical exercise. Now, mechanization and modern conveniences have made most of us lazy. We will take an elevator even to avoid climbing just one flight of stairs. Escalators are seen in almost all modern buildings and department stores, and we will drive our cars to the store even if it is only a block away. We even use remote controls to change channels on our televisions and closed-circuit television to see who's at the door. Lack of exercise has allowed us to become weaker and weaker, but we nonetheless indulge in the great American pastime of *weekend hyperactivity*. During the week, we sit behind a desk or do very little in the way of physical exercise, and then on weekends we catch up with frantic physical exercise. Some executives think nothing of sitting inactive behind a desk for five days and then playing tennis for five hours straight on a sunny Saturday. Others who are overweight, underexercised, and sedentary all year long think nothing of shoveling heavy snow from a long driveway or sidewalk. Is it any wonder that thousands of middle-aged Americans die of heart attacks every winter from just such activity!

Throughout this book I will emphasize the importance of avoiding stress, eating properly, and exercising sensibly and regularly. If we really did these three things, we could prevent 90 percent of all back pain.

PROPER POSTURE

Faulty posture is a major underlying cause of back pain. It can alter the normal curves of the back and put severe stresses on the supporting muscles and ligaments of the spine. A person with round shoulders, a protruding abdomen, and a swayback probably has back pain already, or will most certainly have it in the future. Even the military "West Point" stance (shoulders thrown far back and the chest and derriere sticking out, with a deep swayed curve to the back) constitutes poor posture. The hyperextension of the shoulders and upper spine is abnormal and leads to back pain.

The body has a normal center of gravity. As seen in Fig. 2–1, a line dropped from the level of the ear should cross the

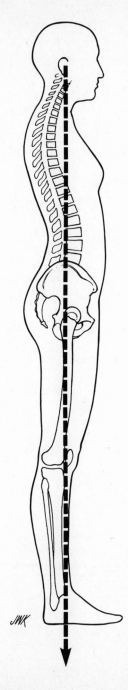

Figure 2–1. The normal center of gravity. A line dropped from the level of the ear should cross the outer tip of the shoulder, middle of the hip, back of the kneecap, and hang in front of the ankle joint. (© Columbia University 1981)

outer tip of the shoulder, middle of the hip, back of the kneecap, and hang in front of the ankle joint. This line represents the center of gravity (CG). If it is too far in front, you will fall forward. If it is too far in back, you will fall backward. If your CG is off, you may assume an abnormal posture, such as round shoulders or a swayback, to try to keep yourself standing upright.

There are five basics to good posture. First of all, it is important to try to stand tall. One good way to remember this is to constantly say to yourself, "Stand tall and look over the fence," as though there were an imaginary fence you were trying to peer over. Some tall people, mostly young women, are so concerned about their excessive height that they tend to slouch to try to make themselves look shorter. A tall woman with good posture is always attractive, while a tall woman who slouches looks unattractive and ends up with back pain as well!

The second basic is head position. Keep your head straight; do not let it jut ahead of the body looking toward the ground. The head should be held back, directly over the shoulders, in a properly balanced position. The average person's head weighs between twenty and twenty-five pounds. Can you imagine balancing a bowling ball, which usually weighs only sixteen pounds, on the end of your finger for very long? That is what we do when we hold our head in front of our spine. We cannot expect the neck muscles to hold this extremely heavy weight in that abnormal position for the entire day—it's almost an impossible feat.

Third, tuck your tummy in and keep it in! The best way to do this is with daily abdominal exercises, which will be discussed in the next chapter. Fourth, tuck in your bottom and hold your rump underneath your pelvis. This should be part of your normal standing posture. If you imagine that there is a silver dollar in the cleft between your buttocks and try to pinch it so that it will not fall out, you will then tighten up the muscles in your derriere and keep your rump tucked properly. Finally, and probably most important of all, never let your lower spine assume a swayback posture. Protruding buttocks and a swayback create a condition known as lordosis, which is very harmful to the vertebrae and spinal nerves in the lower portion of the spine. Lordosis that persists over a period of years can lead to extremely serious spinal problems (see section on spinal stenosis).

NORMAL CURVES OF THE BACK

Early in development, when a baby is carried inside his mother's womb, the spine takes the shape of the letter C. Shortly after birth, the area just below the head and up in the neck, which is called the cervical spine, develops a forward prominence or normal cervical lordosis. Everyone needs this lordosis to keep the head directly over the spine. At the same time, the thoracic spine, which is the area where the ribs attach, develops a posterior curvature, called a kyphosis. This curve can be accurately measured and is normally between 40 and 45 degrees. Finally, the lower portion of the spine, the lumbar area directly above the pelvis, develops what is called the lumbar lordosis. This is a normal forward protrusion of the vertebrae which allows the head and the thoracic spine to be positioned directly over the pelvis (Fig. 2–1). These normal curvatures will help to absorb shock to the spine caused by direct injuries or compressions. If the curves are increased or decreased to too great a degree, excessive stresses are placed on the vertebrae themselves, leading to back pain.

ABNORMAL CURVATURES OF THE BACK

Scoliosis

There are basically three types of abnormal curvatures. They may be seen individually or in combination with each other. The first is called scoliosis. It is a sideways curvature of the spine and can either be to the right or to the left. Scoliosis can occur in either the thoracic region or in the lumbar spine, just above the pelvis. It is extremely common and is seen in approximately 3 to 4 percent of the population in the U.S. Most people with scoliosis have minor curves, and may be totally unaware of them. The only indication of a problem is tilting of the pelvis, with a resultant shortening of the leg on one side. In most cases, scoliosis is insignificant; however, it can occasionally become very severe and require either bracing or spinal surgery for correction.

In the past, scoliosis was mainly seen during great polio epidemics. However, during the last fifteen years polio has been eradicated in major portions of the world. The type of scoliosis seen most commonly today is the genetic form. It is often referred to as idiopathic scoliosis. *Idiopathic* means that we do not know the exact cause; it is a term physicians use to cover up their ignorance. At any rate, one thing we do know about scoliosis is that in most cases it is genetic and inherited through the family tree.

Human genetics are astounding and extremely significant. New life begins at the very instant that the sperm and egg combine. At that instant the new human being is programmed with thousands of genes, the products of certain genetic codes, which will determine once and for all the exact color of the eyes, hair, and skin; body height and muscular proportion; and all other individual characteristics.

Even genetic predisposition to diseases is programmed. We now know that if a woman's mother and grandmother died of breast cancer, her chances of having breast cancer are between 60 percent and 75 percent, no matter what she does during her life. We also know that if a man's father died of either a stroke or coronary artery disease, and this pattern of illness has been present in the family for several generations, his chances of dying of either a stroke or coronary artery disease are about 70 percent. In other words, a great deal of our futures are already determined by the genetic codes we receive at the instant of conception. The only way we can modify these codes is to adapt our bodies and our lives as we grow up. If we take good care of our bodies, they will generally last for a good, long, healthy time. However, if we abuse them, we will suffer for it.

Kyphosis

Kyphosis is a forward curvature of the spine. Normally the thoracic spine, where the ribs are attached, has a kyphosis with an angle of approximately 40 to 45 degrees. Anything in excess of this normal curve is called hyperkyphosis and is usually associated with rounded shoulders and a sunken-chest appearance. Often very tall girls will stand in this posture to try to minimize their height. Certain diseases can cause kyphosis, but they are not very common. Mild forms of hyperkyphosis can be corrected with exercise programs; occasionally braces, which are usually very helpful, are needed as well.

Lordosis

Lordosis has already been mentioned as the term describing the normal forward curve of the cervical and lumbar spine. In the lumbar area, the spine curves forward, thus allowing the thoracic spine to be balanced directly over the pelvis itself. Too much of a curve results in hyperlordosis and puts unusual strains on the lumbar spine, with resulting stresses of the vertebrae themselves and on the small joints between each of the vertebrae in that area.

People with hyperlordosis almost always have a potbelly. As the belly gets larger, the lordosis becomes more exaggerated and the rump sticks out farther. The protruding rump and the belly balance like a cantilevered bridge so that the person doesn't fall forward on his face. As the belly increases in size, the rump grows too; and muscle tone gets weaker and back pain grows more severe. As mentioned in the section on proper posture, it is important to keep the rump tucked underneath the spine so that the pelvis supports the spine and the center of gravity is not displaced in front of the pelvis, which would result in a prominent abdomen and hyperlordosis.

BIOMECHANICS OF THE SPINE

The spine consists of a series of building blocks (the vertebrae) stacked one on top of the other, held together by a marvelously constructed unit consisting of muscles and ligaments, which keep it from collapsing. The ligaments and muscles act in a fashion similar to the guy wires that hold very high radio and television antennas erect. A series of wires on all sides pull in opposite directions, but essentially keep the tower perfectly erect (Fig. 2–2A). If any of these wires become cut or loosened, the tower will sway and collapse toward the opposite side (Fig. 2–2B). Our spines are held erect in the same way by the series of muscles which work *with* (synergistic) and *against* (antagonistic) each other to keep the vertebrae stacked in their precise order (Fig. 2–2C). When the muscles weaken, it is as if a guy wire loosened, and the spinal column starts to sway and bend.

The strongest athlete in the most incredible physical shape can sustain a back injury and be confined in bed for three

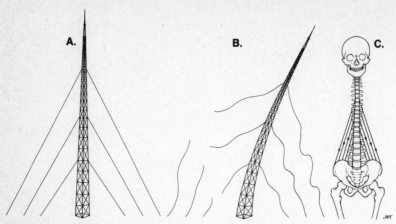

Figure 2–2. The spine is like a radio tower. Notice in A how the tower is held erect because the guy wires pull from all sides and exert a stabilizing force. In B, the wires on one side have been cut and the tower topples toward the other side. C. The human spine is essentially the same as a radio tower; our spinal muscles hold our spine erect through a series of synergistic and antagonistic muscle actions. If these muscles weaken on either side, our spine also tends to weaken and topple like a radio tower. (© Columbia University 1981)

or four weeks. When he finally gets back on his feet, he will be distressed to see how weak his body has become and how lax his muscle tone has gotten in such a short time. We need daily activities and exercises to keep the muscles (guy wires) of the spine in proper tone. Just as we keep a car engine in tune, our spine must be kept in tune by keeping the muscles properly toned so that correct posture is automatic. Any deviation from the normal biomechanics of the spine will cause undue stresses in certain segments of our spinal column and lead to muscle fatigue, muscle spasm, and increasing back pain.

A good friend of mine, during his college years, played varsity football at the University of Wisconsin on a scholarship to finance his education. He is now an extremely successful businessman and has a happy and loving family, but his body is paying the price of many years of severe physical abuses playing football. In essence, he has made a trade-off: He gave up parts of his body for a proper education, an important asset in our society. We all, essentially, make trade-offs in our lives. Sometimes a person becomes a professional athlete. Although he has to abuse his body to reach his goals, the fame and wealth he achieves make it worthwhile to him. The biggest decision you have to make in your life is just how much of a trade-off you are willing to make. If you want to live with a good healthy body, you must put in the time and effort that it takes to keep yourself in good shape; you must exercise daily, eat well-balanced meals, and try to live as stress-free a life as possible.

Three
PREVENTION OF SPINAL PROBLEMS — THE ONE-AUTO-PER-LIFETIME THEORY

Suppose that our government was so concerned about the glut of autos on our highways and in our cities that Congress passed a law restricting each person or family to *one auto per lifetime!* If this were so, we would treat that auto with the greatest care, keeping it serviced, garaged, and waxed to preserve it for every additional mile. After all, we would never be allowed to buy another one.

Actually, we are only given one body per lifetime. Why do we abuse it with stresses, improper diet, and lack of exercise? We treat our bodies most disrespectfully—we smoke, drink, live at too fast a pace, and deprive ourselves of sleep. We act as though we can make a trade-in every three years or fifty thousand miles. Unfortunately, this is not so. Although we rarely treat our body with the same care we show the family car, when something happens to it we run to our doctor and say, "Give me a pill or a shot, and fix it up, Doc!"

If people would only take care of their bodies as well as they take care of their cars, doctors' offices would be less crowded, and millions of hours of misery and back pain could be prevented. Remember, your body must last a lifetime—treat it well!

WEIGHT CONTROL

Diet and Activity—Calories Do Count!

Some years ago a book came out entitled *Calories Don't Count.* Nothing could be further from the truth. People flocked to buy the book, even though authorities around the world assure us that calories do count and that every single piece of food we take into our bodies contains some calories. The average person requires only two thousand to three thousand calories a day. Naturally, the number of calories you need depends on exactly how many calories you burn. Taking in calories is the same as adding gasoline to your car's gas tank. If the gas tank only holds fifteen gallons, and you try to put twenty gallons into the tank, you're going to spill some gas on the pavement. Our bodies do not just spill over excess calories, but turn them into fat and extra weight.

Most adolescents burn up a tremendous amount of calories because they are extremely active, as any parent knows. Young people run and play a great deal and burn up many calories with nervous energy. Children can eat enormous quantities of food and still not put on weight. With age, however, especially after the age of thirty-five, body proportions change and the nice physiques of youth slowly start to shift and settle into shapes that are less pleasurable. Muscle tone tends to diminish and most of us get rather soggy in the abdomen and wider in the thighs and buttocks. This is when we need to develop a tremendous awareness of the effect of calories. Actually, we should begin watching in our early twenties.

As our lives become more complicated and the stresses of raising a family take their toll, many adults begin to drink and eat excessively. They also become more sedentary and begin watching television for long periods while nibbling away at high-caloric snacks. If most of us were to really keep an accurate count of all the calories we take in during a twenty-four-hour period, we would be astounded to see that we far exceed the two thousand to three thousand calories we need. Since *calories do count* and certain foods contain tremendous numbers of calories (especially alcohol), we must learn to eat foods that nourish us most and yet do not turn us into globs of fat. Calorie counters are available at practically every drugstore. With brief reference to these booklets, we can rapidly learn which foods give us the greatest amount of energy value and how many calories they contain.

Some foods actually contribute no calories to the body. Celery is an example—it is mostly water, and the action of chewing it burns up so many calories that it is actually a *negative*-caloric food even though it is filling. Other foods like ice cream or whipped cream on a cake will add hundreds of calories to the diet.

It is also important to be aware of the caloric requirements of various activities. For instance, sawing wood for an hour burns up between 400 and 600 calories. Sewing burns up only 10 to 30 calories per hour, while sweeping or dusting burns up between 80 and 130 calories per hour. Walking at 2 miles per hour burns up 200 calories; a brisker walk of 4 miles per hour burns up 350 calories per hour. Running burns up between 800 and 1,000 calories per hour, while dancing burns up only 200 to 400 calories per hour. Although wrestling is a strenuous exercise (it burns up between 900 and 1,000 calories per hour), it is rather impractical as a daily exercise. Probably the best exercise of all is swimming. The crawl stroke burns up between 700 to 900 calories per hour and the breast and back strokes burn between 350 and 650 calories per hour. By referring to caloric and exercise guides, we can quickly assess the amount of calories and exercise we need to stay in proper trim. By weighing yourself at least twice a week, you can keep your weight under control. Don't weigh yourself every day because daily flunctuations in weight of between one and three pounds are common.

DOS AND DON'TS FOR SPINAL HEALTH

Although sitting is one of the most common positions assumed during our waking hours, it also happens to be one of the most stressful postures for our backs. It is important to choose a chair that provides a firm support, especially in the lumbar region (Fig. 3–1). The feet should be slightly elevated; they can be placed on a raised board or stool under the desk. If you are

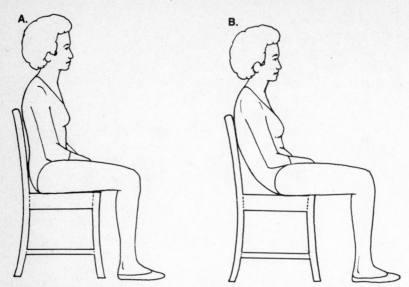

Figure 3–1. A. Illustration of the proper way to sit in a straight-back chair. B. Illustrates the slouching posture most people acquire, which ultimately leads to muscle weakness and back pain.

sewing, use a small footstool. A woman who is ironing or preparing dinner at the kitchen counter should put one foot on a low footstool because this flattens out the lumbar spine and gets rid of lumbar hyperlordosis, thus reducing spinal stress (Fig. 3–2A and B). The brass rail provided in most saloons serves the same purpose. If people stand at a bar and are comfortable they will buy more drinks and keep the saloon keeper in business. The brass rail reduces the stress on the lumbar spine, thereby reducing lumbar muscle fatigue. At the same time, the alcohol intake also has an anesthetic effect on any muscle spasm or back pain, thereby working in conjunction with the brass rail to turn the customer into a happy patron (Fig. 3–2C). It is important to keep one leg elevated slightly when you are engaged in any type of activity that requires prolonged standing. It is also important to occasionally get up, stretch, and walk around to relieve muscular strain. This can be most helpful when you are confined to an airplane seat for a long period of time.

    In the past few years plastic credit cards have thickened wallets considerably, and many men now have prominent

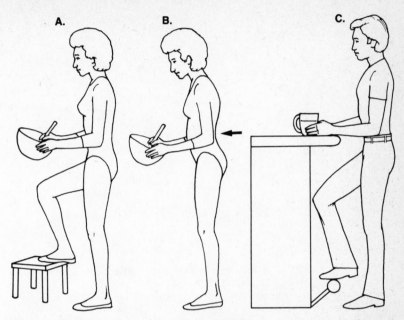

Figure 3–2. The proper way to work at home. If you elevate one leg on a small stool, you flatten out your spine and provide proper spinal mechanics, causing the head to remain directly over the pelvis and decreasing muscle fatigue. This is also helpful when ironing. C. The reason most taverns have a brass rail at the bar is to flatten the lumbar spine to reduce swayback. This makes for happier patrons.

bulges in their hip pockets. When a man sits for prolonged periods, his bulging wallet presses directly on his sciatic nerve on that side and can cause severe sciatica (leg pain). Wallets should be thinned down or carried in the inside coat pocket or elsewhere to avoid this problem.

Another helpful tip involves the proper way to pick up objects. It is important not to bend from the waist, but to *squat down,* keeping the back straight. This reduces pressure on the lumbar region, which is, of course, the site of most backache (Fig. 3–3). Poor sleeping posture is one of the major causes of low back pain. It is important to use a firm mattress; many people who suffer from low back pain tell me that they are most comfortable when they lie on the bedroom floor. When they are in a hotel with a soft mattress, they often order a bed board under the mattress or sleep directly on the floor.

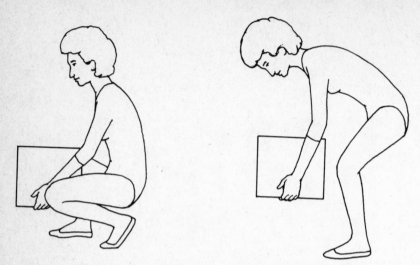

Figure 3–3. The correct and incorrect ways to lift up a heavy object. When squatting, most stresses are taken up by the thigh and abdominal muscles. If a patient bends over, the stresses are taken up by the spine only, and could severely injure ligaments and muscles.

Some people find that sleeping on a heated water bed or a bed filled with gel is very soothing to the back. These beds are not for everyone, and you should test them before investing in one. If you are considering a water or a gel bed, spend a few nights in motels that advertise these types of beds and find out for yourself just how comfortable they are. Some back patients of mine think they are great; others find that they aggravate back pain and prefer an extremely firm mattress, with a bed board underneath, in some cases. Remember, what works for one person will not necessarily work for another.

A bed board is a solid sheet of plywood which should be five-eighths inch to three-quarters inch thick. It can be inserted directly between the innerspring and the mattress itself, and is available at any lumber store. You can call ahead to hotels and request a bed board, thus saving yourself a night of agony on a mattress that is too soft. If you are very tall, phone ahead and ask for an extra-long bed. Most motels and hotels have these and will be happy to accommodate you. Cramming a long body into a short bed for eight hours can lead to days of agony.

When sleeping, try to lie on the side and bend your knees (the fetal position). Many people find that putting a small pillow between the knees makes them even more comfortable. Sleeping with a pillow that is not too bulky under the head and a pillow between the knees in a side position can be most comfortable. You should always avoid lying directly on your belly because that position increases lumbar swayback (lordosis) and will contribute to increasing back pain (Fig. 3–4). Our vertebrae are not intended to be arched backward the way they are when we sleep in that position. It's the same as if you were trying to open a door in the opposite direction from which the hinges open. If you force the door, the hinges will eventually come loose and rip off the wall.

If you like to sleep directly on your back, a small pillow between the head and neck, as well as a small pillow under the knees, will make you more comfortable. Most of you, of course, roll around during your sleep; sleep studies have shown that you change positions during the night between twenty and thirty times. With a little bit of subconscious effort, however, you can learn to avoid the most harmful position, lying on your tummy, even while asleep. (If you live with someone, ask your sleeping partner to awaken you if you accidentally roll over on your tummy).

High-heeled shoes are also bad for your back. They throw the spine out of line and change the center of gravity by tilting the pelvis forward and increasing lumbar swayback. Many women, especially those in the working world, feel they

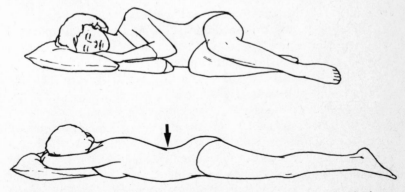

Figure 3–4. The proper way to sleep. When sleeping on the side, the knees can be pulled up and the lower spine flattened. When sleeping on your tummy, spinal swayback is increased in the lower spine, especially if the mattress is too soft, leading to backache the next day.

must wear high heels. A sensible heel—that is no more than two or two and a half inches in height—can be fairly comfortable for most of the day, especially if the diameter of the heel is thick enough to provide a proper platform for body weight. Four- and five-inch stiletto heels are extremely harmful for the back and should not be worn for prolonged periods. Although they make a woman's legs look lovely by accentuating the calf and thigh muscles, high heels are not sensible or comfortable, and should be avoided if at all possible.

Driving long distances can cause extreme pain in the lower back. New, better-designed car seats offered by certain manufacturers to replace your present car seats are worth the investment if you have chronic back pain. Auto manufacturers are becoming more aware of the need for proper spinal support and comfort during prolonged driving. A much greater effort is now being made to see that auto seats are comfortable and that they orthopaedically support the spine.

When you have back pain, it is important to stop and get out of your car about every hour for a cup of coffee or a snack so you can move your body around and relieve muscle fatigue. It is also important to position your car seat forward as much as possible so that your knees are bent (Fig. 3–5). This position reduces swayback in your lower spine. A small cushion placed in the small of your back will be most helpful. Occasionally changing the tilt in the car seat will change the angle of the spine and provide further relief. Sports cars with extremely low seats that cause the legs to extend practically straight out in front of you are probably the most harmful designs for the spine. If you are prone to prolonged backaches and your auto trip will be more than a few hours, you are probably much better off flying and then renting a car if necessary.

Social affairs can be a time of great aggravation for the chronic back pain sufferer. When you are at a cocktail party, don't stand in one position for too long. Move around the room and talk to various people. Again, if it is possible, raise one leg on a small footstool while talking so you flatten out the lower spine and make yourself more comfortable. Shifting the weight from one foot to the other also helps relieve stress in the lower back, and sitting down for brief periods will help distribute lumbar spine pressures.

Women should avoid extremely tight jeans and tight girdles. When they are worn for long periods of time, especially

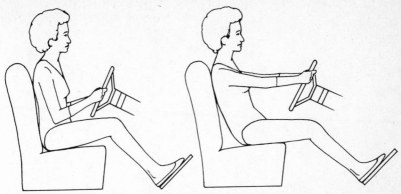

Figure 3–5. When driving, always sit with your seat as close to the steering wheel as is comfortable and with your knees slightly elevated to flatten out the swayback in your lower spine. Sitting with the legs out, as is done in most sports cars, usually produces fatigue in the lower spinal muscles.

over a period of many years, the abdominal muscles tend to become soft. The girdle holds the belly in, usurping the role of the abdominal muscles. Our spinal muscles also weaken after years of girdle wear. A woman may find she is unable to go without a girdle at all because she is now "married" to the support the girdle provides. It is much better to improve your muscle tone to keep the belly flat. Tight girdles also can lead to varicose veins in the legs because they prevent the veins from returning blood from the legs to the heart.

People who need to carry cases of material or gear on their shoulders in the course of their work should see to it that the loads are well-balanced on both shoulders. If you cannot distribute the weight evenly, you should carry such parcels in alternate hands so that the weight is shifted from side to side and excessive stresses are not borne for too long a period on any one side.

Basically, you should stand up straight and keep your rump and pelvis tucked under your lumbar spine. Keep your shoulders back comfortably and your abdomen pulled in, but try to be as *relaxed* as possible. A good test of posture is to back up against a wall and put your head and your heels against it. Then try to flatten out the small of your back so that it practically touches the wall. Walk away from the wall in this position, and you will have the position of most comfort for prolonged standing (Fig 3–6).

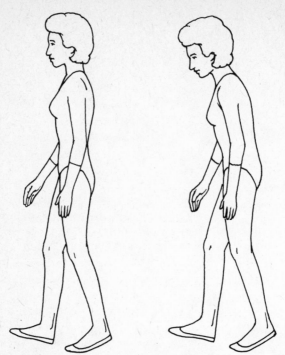

Figure 3–6. Proper and improper ways to walk. Always stand tall, tuck in your tummy, and flatten out your swayback by pushing your pelvis forward.

EXERCISES TO PREVENT BACK PROBLEMS: THE FIVE KPEs (KEIM PREVENTIVE EXERCISES)

For the last twenty-five years I have done regular spine exercises daily. *I am not an exercise nut* and frankly do not enjoy doing exercises. Some people are physical types and routinely do all kinds of exercises, but most of us, unfortunately, are not. I realize how difficult it is to get up out of bed, a soft chair, or to come home after a hard day's work and try to make yourself exercise. Nothing could be more difficult! I am basically a morning person and have found that if I set my clock to go off just fifteen minutes earlier in the morning, I can do my five basic preventive exercises for low back pain daily. This routine has kept me in excellent physical muscle tone, and I have never had a serious problem with my back, although I lead a most strenuous life.

I have taught my five preventive exercises, which are referred to as the KPEs (Keim Preventive Exercises), to literally hundreds of patients and can honestly say that if they are done exactly as I describe, on a *daily basis*, almost everyone will show a marked improvement. The idea is to put your body through a series of repetitious physical activities and to keep increasing the repetitions as the months and years go by so that each day you put the ligaments, tendons, muscles, and cardiovascular system through a proper coordination program that maintains your physical fitness. A well-trained athlete who has a serious fall will probably not be injured, while even a minor fall can cause a serious injury in a middle-aged person who is overweight and underexercised. These injuries can be avoided by doing the daily preventive exercises I outline.

Before you start any exercise program, if you are over the age of thirty-five, you should check with your physician to make certain that you do not have any serious ailments that could be made worse by exercising. If you have a cardiac problem or other physical condition that restricts exercise, you should discuss this in detail with your physician before undertaking this program.

Once you start your exercise program, never skip a day unless you are extremely ill or a catastrophe occurs. The whole value of these exercises rests on *daily* use. Fortunately, it only takes about twelve to fifteen minutes to do them. They can be done by both men and women alike, and they can be performed in the confines of your bedroom or even in a motel room if you are traveling. They can also be done on the beach or even in the doctor's locker room after surgery! When I first started doing my exercises in the doctor's locker room at the Columbia-Presbyterian Medical Center, my colleagues looked at me with amazement. In fact, I was the subject of many snide comments and jokes. Over the years, however, many of my colleagues have begun exercising too and are impressed with their improved stamina and energy—plus they are extremely pleased with their trimmer physiques.

Remember to avoid fatigue, which can cause undue soreness and muscle stiffness. The old adage that says you must exercise until it hurts is absolutely wrong; it only applies to people who are professional weight lifters and are trying to increase their muscle bulk. The average person should exercise within the limits of comfort. You should do the exercises slowly and gradually, trying to relax as much as possible. At the same time, try to limber yourself up and stretch your muscles out so that you develop more strength and flexibility. Get yourself in the proper frame of mind to do your exercises. You must absolutely reserve fifteen minutes a day as a "holy time," set aside just for you. We set aside time three times a day in which to eat and nourish our bodies. We also set aside time in which to take care of our bathroom and body functions. We waste hours in front of television sets and spend hours talking with friends and family. Certainly fifteen minutes a day to spend on our bodies is not too much to ask for the incredible rewards that follow.

Never delay your exercises because you feel that you are so rushed that you just can't possibly do them. I found long ago that if I skip my exercises in the morning and do not do them before noon, I am too tired by the time I get home at seven or eight o'clock in the evening and have my supper. I have learned to do them right after I wake up. I usually turn on the television and watch the morning news while I exercise. After my fifteen-minute KPE program, I hop into the shower and proceed with my day.

Perform the exercises slowly and smoothly. Try to avoid jerky movements and try not to strain yourself by doing too many at one time. Last, never do more repetitions than you are ready for. When you start with the five KPEs, do them at a *low enough frequency so that you do not hurt yourself.* Some years ago, while I was doing my exercises and was up to many repetitions with all five of them, I developed a severe cold and the flu and found myself in bed for about six days. When I recovered I tried to return to the rate and frequency of exercise I had reached before I had become bedridden. I found it extremely difficult to do them, and I injured my muscles and had severe soreness and ligament tenderness for several weeks. (Even doctors do stupid things occasionally!) You must always resist the urge to do too many repetitions of any of the five exercises at any one time. You must work your way up slowly, and if for some reason you are forced to miss several days, you must drop back several levels and reduce the frequency of the repetitions until you are again comfortable and can slowly move ahead on a daily basis. You should start out doing only a certain basic number of repetitions depending on your age and general physical condition at the time you start the KPEs. Then, every *third* day, increase the repetitions by only one or two in each of the five exercises so that eventually (after about six months) you will reach a plateau that is proper and reasonable for your age and body type. The secret of the KPEs is to do them *daily* and *progress slowly!*

I now do two hundred jumping jacks as exercise number one, sixty toe touches as exercise number two, sixty-five push-ups as exercise number three, seventy-five sit-ups as exercise number four, and three series of two hundred steps running in place, interrupted by fifteen scissors jumps. The entire program takes about fifteen minutes. It is important to stay within that time framework, as this increases your heart and breathing

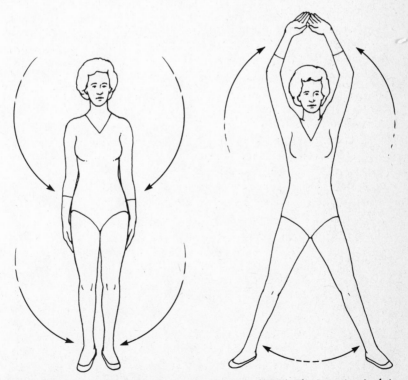

Figure 3–7. The first Keim Preventive Exercise (KPE). The jumping jack is well known to everyone and should be done smoothly and gracefully.

rates to the point where it slightly stresses these organs and keeps them in proper tone. I must emphasize, however, that it has taken me almost twenty years to get up to this level of activities and to this number of repetitions. As I get older, I will have to cut down the repetitions slightly because my muscle bulk will deteriorate with age.

In succession, I will describe each of the five KPEs, referring to the appropriate illustrations.

The *first KPE* (Fig. 3–7) is a *jumping jack.* This exercise should be done rhythmically and smoothly, without sudden jerking movements, and should be started rather slowly until you are properly warmed up. The average person, age thirty, who is starting to do these exercises probably should do no more than twenty *at the most* for the first week, and then slowly, every second or third day, add another repetition.

The *second KPE* (Fig. 3–8) is a toe-touch exercise with the feet together. Bend directly forward at first, then swing six inches to the left of the left foot and touch the floor; next swing

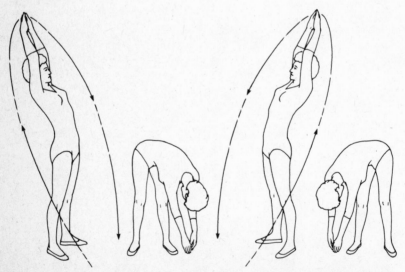

Figure 3–8. The second Keim Preventive Exercise (KPE) is a toe touch to six inches on either side of the feet. It is important that you keep your hands together and sway in a gentle arc from side to side as you perform the exercise. First do a series of exercises from left to right, and then continue the same exercises until you do an equal number from right to left.

six inches to the right of the right foot, and touch the floor. Swing and arch the back around in a general circle. Alternate the direction by doing some from left to right and then doing an equal number from right to left. At first you will find it extremely difficult to touch the ground in front of you without bending your knees, especially if you are not used to doing any exercises. If you can't reach, it is permissible to spread your legs slightly and only touch the ground in front of you at first. This will suffice until you have stretched out the ligaments and muscles around your pelvis and in back of your knees. If you can already touch the floor with your knees straight, you can probably start by doing the toe-touch exercise five times from left to right and five times from right to left. You should not increase the repetitions for at least a week to ten days, and then very slowly—every third or fourth day—increase by one repetition from left to right and another from right to left.

The *third KPE* (Fig. 3-9) is the pushup. If you feel particularly weak when starting the exercise program, do the pushups in the kneeling position, sometimes referred to as the woman's pushup. (Fig. 3–9A) These are much easier because you are not supporting the entire lower trunk on your toes, and require less strength than the routine male pushup. I would recommend that at first you try doing only four or five pushups. Continue these every day for the first week to ten days, and then slowly—every third day—increase by an additional repetition. Change from the kneeling-type pushup to a regular routine pushup as soon as possible, but cut back the repetitions to only four or five, at most, and slowly increase as you get stronger (Fig. 3–9C).

The *fourth KPE* (Fig. 3–10) consists of a sit-up. It is important to keep your knees bent so that the forces used in sitting up are mainly contractions of the abdominal muscles. Some people find it impossible to do sit-ups without hooking their toes under some stationary object. (Be certain that the object cannot topple or fall over on you; use something heavy, such as the edge of a bed or a heavy dresser.) Excellent home slant boards or gym devices are also available at extremely modest prices that have straps under which you can hook your toes. Generally, most people find it is easiest to do the sit-up at first with their hands clasped behind their head. They then bend forward until they touch their knees with their elbows. This is a

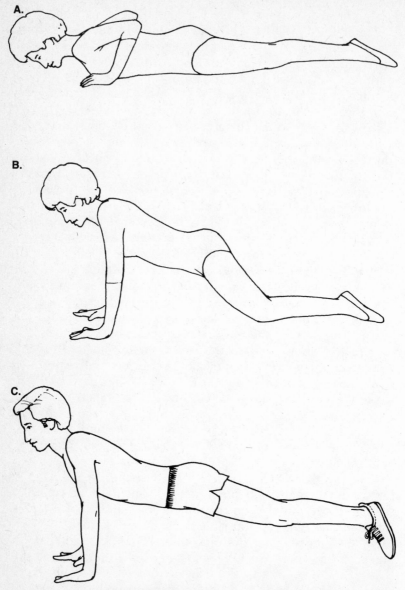

Figure 3–9. The third Keim Preventive Exercise (KPE) is the pushup. In A and B, you see what is commonly known as a woman's pushup, where the person remains on the knees. However, it is a much more helpful exercise to try to do the man's pushup, where you balance on your toes in the extended arm position.

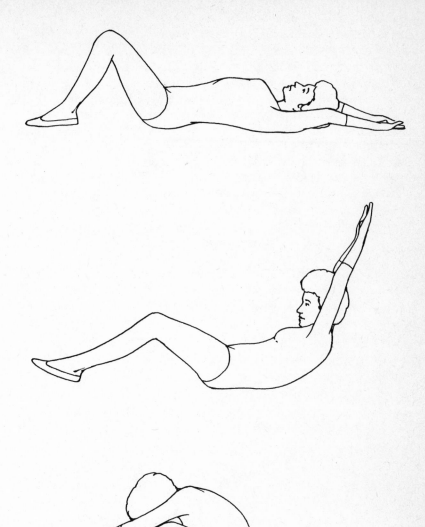

Figure 3–10. The fourth Keim Preventive Exercise (KPE) is the sit-up, keeping the arms extended and level with the ears. It is sometimes necessary to hook your toes under some heavy, stationary object and to keep the knees slightly bent. This stresses the abdominal muscles and is excellent for flattening the tummy.

perfectly acceptable way to start. Eventually, as your muscle tone increases, it is best to keep the arms stretched out and *behind* the level of your ears, because this increases the leverage on the trunk and makes it more difficult to sit up, thus making the abdominal muscles work harder. I would recommend that you begin with hands clasped behind your ears; do only five or six sit-ups to start. Increase the repetitions (after the first week to ten days) about every third day by one repetition. I usually do fifty of these sit-ups with my arms stretched out behind my ears, and then do twenty-five more sit-ups with my hands clasped across my abdomen. These are easier to do, and strengthen the lower lumbar and abdominal muscles even more. They increase your muscle tone and help to keep your tummy flat. If you wish, you can do some sit-up exercises with your arms behind your ears and some with your hands clasped over your tummy.

The *fifth KPE* (Fig. 3–11) is simple. It consists of running in place, and is somewhat boring. If you watch television or even watch yourself in a full-length mirror, you will find that it is

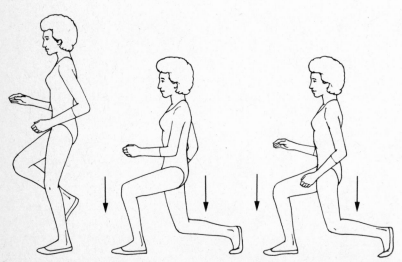

Figure 3–11. The fifth Keim Preventive Exercise (KPE) is running in place, followed by a series of scissors jumps, which are illustrated here. The scissors jump consists of a straddle jump with the legs apart and alternating the legs in the squatting position. This exercise is not only for lower spinal muscles, but also for the thigh muscles.

easier to do. It helps to watch your reflection in a mirror to see how well you are performing your exercises and to improve your timing. When running in place, it is important that you pick up your feet at least six inches above the floor. Generally, as I mentioned, I do three series of two hundred steps running in place and then fifteen scissors jumps, which each end up with a deep knee squat. This will be very difficult to do in the beginning, and I would recommend that you run only fifty steps at first and instead of doing a deep knee squat, just do three scissors jumps. After eight or ten days you can slowly increase the repetitions by adding five or ten steps every fourth or fifth day; increase the scissors jumps by one or two as time goes on. I repeat, the secret of the KPEs is to do them *daily* and progress slowly!

As mentioned before, remember *not to try to achieve too much too soon.* It will take you probably six months to a year to get to a proper level of exercise for your age. Once you have gotten there you will know it, and you can then stay at the maintenance level for the rest of your life—on a *daily* basis.

Secondly, be sure to do your exercises *every single day.* If you look forward to doing the exercises because you know that they help you and try not to procrastinate, you will enjoy doing them more and they will work wonders for your confidence and your body. I have learned that the best way not to procrastinate is just to start doing them! The minute I start thinking about doing them I usually can find about 220 reasons why I really shouldn't do them; but once I start the exercises, I usually have no difficulty finishing. With the help of the five KPEs you will, hopefully, never need to do the exercises described in the next section for people who already have back pain (the PREs).

As you progress through your exercise program and the first six months go by, you will be pleasantly surprised to see how much more attractive your physique becomes.

EXERCISES IF YOU ALREADY HAVE BACK PAIN: THE SIX PREs (PAIN RELIEVING EXERCISES)

Most people who have back pain that does not involve pain radiating down the back of the leg have a form of lumbar strain. This can be either acute (of sudden onset and short duration) or chronic (injury that has lasted for months or years). If acute back pain is really severe, you should stay in bed, take warm (not hot) tub baths at least twice a day, use a heating pad or a hydrocollator, get adequate sleep on a firm mattress with a bed board, and see a physician for proper diagnosis and medication.

If you have chronic back pain, you must usually lose weight and improve your posture, as well as use a firm mattress with a bed board, do the PREs, and participate in regular sports activities compatible with your age and physique.

You should *never* do exercises when you are experiencing acute low back pain; you should be in bed resting! However, when you have chronic back pain and general muscle aches, the Pain-Relieving Exercises (PREs), *done daily,* can be most helpful. These exercises are a distillation of those offered by many physical therapists and doctors throughout the world.

The *first PRE* (Fig. 3–12): Lie on your back with your arms on your chest and your knees bent and tuck your tail by pressing the small of the back to the floor while tightening the abdominal muscles. This tilts the pelvis, flattens excessive lumbar lordosis or swayback, and brings the pelvis directly underneath the lumbar vertebrae. The position is held for a count of ten. Relax, then repeat the exercise. At first do three or four repetitions daily. Every second or third day increase the repetitions by one.

For the *second PRE*, lie on your back with your arms at your sides and your knees bent. Draw your knees up to the chest. This action helps flatten excessive swayback and strengthen lumbar and abdominal muscles. Again, the exercise should be repeated only two or three times at first, and the repetitions increased every second or third day if pain is not severe. If any of the exercises aggravates the pain, stop and consult your doctor.

For the *third PRE*, lie on your back with your knees bent and your arms folded on your chest. Sit up, using the abdominal muscles. The arms can then be stretched forward to help you keep your balance. For this exercise it is sometimes helpful to hook your toes underneath a heavy, stationary object, such as a bed.

The *fourth PRE* is a forward knee-flexion exercise. Begin in the typical runners' starting position, and press forward several times, flexing your knee and bringing your abdomen to your thigh. This action not only strengthens the lower extremity muscles, but stretches out the spinal and hamstring muscles.

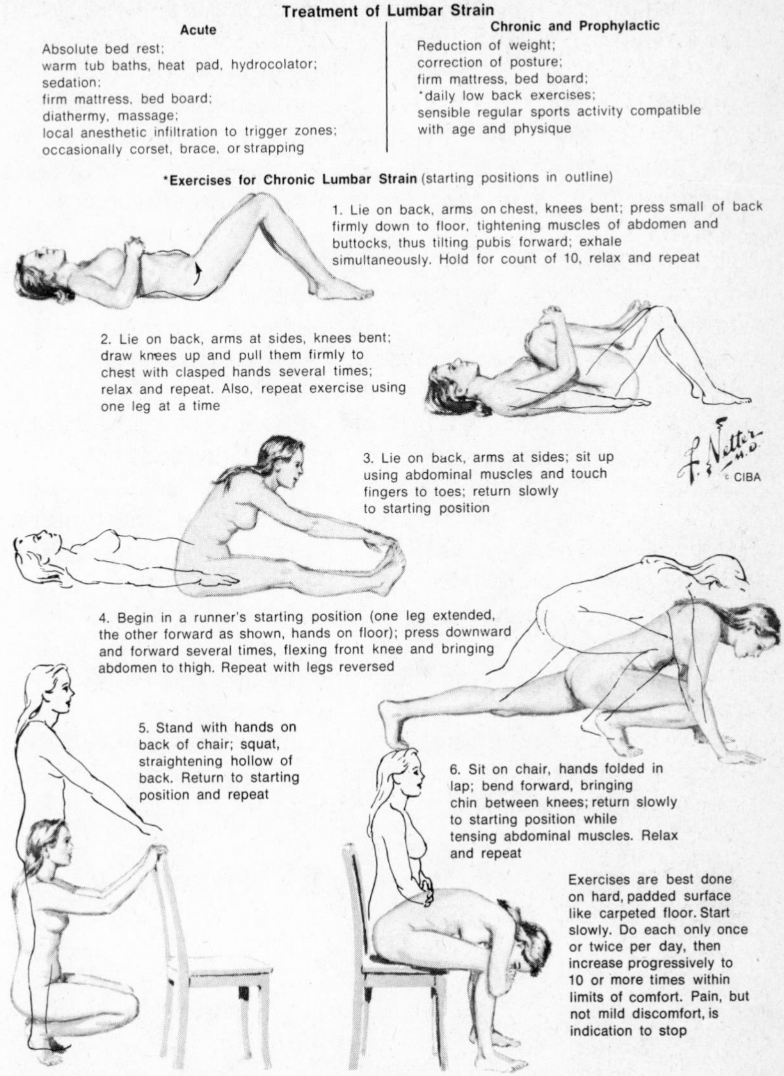

Treatment of Lumbar Strain

Acute

Absolute bed rest;
warm tub baths, heat pad, hydrocolator;
sedation;
firm mattress, bed board;
diathermy, massage;
local anesthetic infiltration to trigger zones;
occasionally corset, brace, or strapping

Chronic and Prophylactic

Reduction of weight;
correction of posture;
firm mattress, bed board;
*daily low back exercises;
sensible regular sports activity compatible
with age and physique

*Exercises for Chronic Lumbar Strain (starting positions in outline)

1. Lie on back, arms on chest, knees bent; press small of back firmly down to floor, tightening muscles of abdomen and buttocks, thus tilting pubis forward; exhale simultaneously. Hold for count of 10, relax and repeat

2. Lie on back, arms at sides, knees bent; draw knees up and pull them firmly to chest with clasped hands several times; relax and repeat. Also, repeat exercise using one leg at a time

3. Lie on back, arms at sides; sit up using abdominal muscles and touch fingers to toes; return slowly to starting position

4. Begin in a runner's starting position (one leg extended, the other forward as shown, hands on floor); press downward and forward several times, flexing front knee and bringing abdomen to thigh. Repeat with legs reversed

5. Stand with hands on back of chair; squat, straightening hollow of back. Return to starting position and repeat

6. Sit on chair, hands folded in lap; bend forward, bringing chin between knees; return slowly to starting position while tensing abdominal muscles. Relax and repeat

Exercises are best done on hard, padded surface like carpeted floor. Start slowly. Do each only once or twice per day, then increase progressively to 10 or more times within limits of comfort. Pain, but not mild discomfort, is indication to stop

Figure 3–12. The six Pain-Relieving Exercises (PREs). These exercises can be most helpful once you have pain. They should be done every day on a regular basis, and the instructions listed along with them should be followed exactly. If they increase pain in any way, you should reduce the repetitions or stop altogether. Any time that the pain is markedly increased, consult your doctor. (Copyright © 1980, CIBA Pharmaceutical Company)

Reverse legs with every other repetition. Again, these exercises should only be done four or five times when you start the program and increased by one repetition every second or third day.

✓ For the *fifth PRE*, stand with your hands on the back of a chair. Then squat down, keeping your back as straight as possible. This exercise can be done four or five times to start with and again increased by one repetition every second or third day.

✓Begin the *sixth PRE* sitting in a chair with your hands folded in your lap. Then bend forward so that your head is hanging just slightly below your knees. This action tenses the abdominal muscles and also helps strengthen the spinal muscles.

In general, the PREs should be done on a hard, padded surface or a bedroom carpet. Start slowly! The PREs should be done at least once a day. If you feel up to it, you can do them twice a day, first in the morning and again in the evening. Increase repetitions progressively to thirty or more times *within the limits of your comfort*. Pain that seems to be getting worse is an indication to stop; however, mild discomfort is normal and to be expected.

Like the KPEs, the PREs should be done *daily!* If you have experienced back pain, these exercises will help reduce it. You can then combine these six exercises with the five KPEs for a program of eleven superb exercises that not only prevent pain, but also give you excellent muscle tone!

A SIMPLIFIED PROGRAM OF BACK CONTROL FOR BETTER SPINAL HEALTH

If you do the five KPEs and the six PREs daily, control stress, and have a good diet, you can generally ensure that your back will stay normal and relatively pain-free. This simplified program will control your back and keep it strengthened and *stop back problems before they start!* A few hours spent preventing spinal disorders will save many hours of bed rest and traction. If you are willing to make this minimal investment of time and energy, your spine will grow stronger daily. The exercises described seek to eliminate excessive swayback or lumbar lordosis. Swayback posture is one of the major causes of back pain and should be avoided at all times.

Four

WHAT THINGS CAN GO WRONG WITH YOUR BACK?

DIAGNOSIS AND CLASSIFICATION

In this chapter, the major things that can go wrong with your back will be reviewed. Many unfamiliar medical terms will appear, but I will try to break them down and simplify them. However, for the sake of completeness, most conditions will be mentioned and will be grouped in specific medical categories.

MECHANICAL CAUSES OF BACK PAIN

Mechanical causes of back pain can be divided into what I call *intrinsic* or *extrinsic* causes. Intrinsic factors are those strictly associated with muscle strength and postural tone, while extrinsic ones are the result of conditions in the body which are outside of the spine itself, such as pelvic tumors, kidney or hip disease.

Intrinsic Causes of Back Pain

Poor muscle tone, which often results in muscular strains and ligament sprains, is one intrinsic cause of back pain; postural imbalance and weakness are others. For good posture the head should be held erect with the chest out, abdomen in, back flat, and the buttocks tucked under the spine. A person with good

43

posture will rarely have back problems. However, the patients who come into my office usually hold their heads forward; their chests are flat, the abdomen protrudes, they have a swayback (with buttocks out), and are overweight with terrible muscle tone (Fig. 4–1). They did not get this way overnight—it took many years of soft living and overeating! Now they are paying the piper with back pain. The condition can be reversed, but not without a serious *daily* effort to lose weight, exercise, and adopt a new posture.

Another type of intrinsically caused back pain is caused by inflammation and tenderness of the muscles and of the sheets that envelop the muscles, the fascia. This inflammation affects middle-aged persons and is called myofascitis. Firm, localized, tender, and nodular deposits develop in the muscle sheaths on both sides of the spine, causing very severe, ill-defined back pain. The pain is often initiated and aggravated by overuse of these muscles. Exposure to cold and drafts is particularly likely to initiate the back pain. Usually this type of pain occurs in patients who have poor muscle tone to begin with and have tried to do something strenuous. The sudden burst of activity brings on a muscular spasm. The nodules can be injected with pain-killing agents or cortisone-type drugs to relieve pain. Proper posture, weight reduction, and regular exercise are mandatory for relief.

Unstable lumbar vertebrae are another intrinsic cause of back pain. In this condition a vertebra, usually in the lumbar spine, shifts backward and forward on the vertebrae above and below it. Back pain is severe because the nerve roots that emerge from between the vertebrae are pinched, giving rise to nerve-root pain. The third and fourth, or the fourth and fifth lumbar vertebrae are most frequently involved. Displacement of the vertebrae is usually forward and occurs when bending forward, reaching, or leaning too far backward. The condition can be best detected on X rays taken while the patient is bending forward or straightening out completely. The condition can also be detected on movie-type X rays (ciné). Patients with unstable vertebrae usually show marked improvement with spinal exercises and brief use of a corset. Surgery is not often indicated because patients with unstable vertebrae usually tend to have degenerative arthritic changes in their entire spine and surgery rarely offers a permanent cure. However, when the pain does not

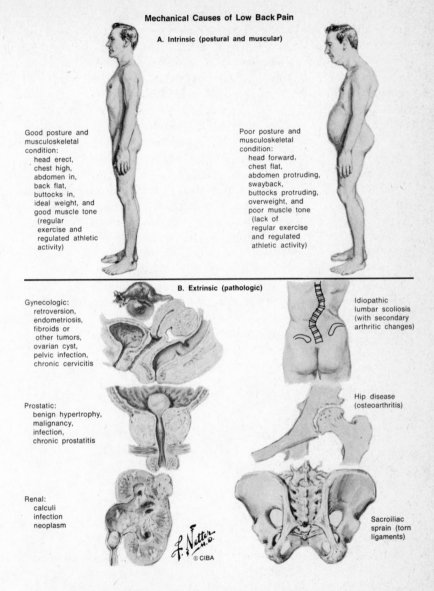

Mechanical Causes of Low Back Pain

A. Intrinsic (postural and muscular)

Good posture and musculoskeletal condition:
head erect,
chest high,
abdomen in,
back flat,
buttocks in,
ideal weight, and
good muscle tone
(regular
exercise and
regulated athletic
activity)

Poor posture and musculoskeletal condition:
head forward,
chest flat,
abdomen protruding,
swayback,
buttocks protruding,
overweight, and
poor muscle tone
(lack of
regular exercise
and regulated
athletic activity)

B. Extrinsic (pathologic)

Gynecologic:
retroversion,
endometriosis,
fibroids or
other tumors,
ovarian cyst,
pelvic infection,
chronic cervicitis

Idiopathic
lumbar scoliosis
(with secondary
arthritic changes)

Prostatic:
benign hypertrophy,
malignancy,
infection,
chronic prostatitis

Hip disease
(osteoarthritis)

Renal:
calculi
infection
neoplasm

Sacroiliac
sprain (torn
ligaments)

Figure 4–1. Mechanical causes of back pain. A. Intrinsic causes (postural and muscular). B. Extrinsic causes—those due to pain referred from other parts of the body. Examples are shown of problems in the female organs, prostate gland, or kidneys; or secondary to scoliosis, hip disease, and ligament sprain. (Copyright © 1980, CIBA Pharmaceutical Company)

respond to nonoperative treatment, occasionally a surgical fusion that welds the offending vertebra to the one above and the one below it can provide lasting relief.

The effect of increased swayback or hyperlordosis has been discussed previously. Poor posture is an extremely important mechanical cause of low back pain. With age, most people's abdomens and buttocks protrude as a result of a decrease in muscle activity and an increase in body weight. Poor posture begets even poorer posture, until eventually the pelvis is no longer underneath the spine and cannot support it. A shearing effect takes place as all of the weight above the lumbar spine is directed to the front of the center of gravity, and marked structural and stressful changes occur in the lumbar spine. The hyperlordosis (increased swayback) narrows the little foramina (windows) of the vertebrae where the nerve roots exit (Fig. 4–2) and causes nerve root entrapment, with severe pain across the buttocks and down the lower extremities. Eventually, narrowing may lead to spinal stenosis. The symptoms mimic those of a herniated disc, and the disc disorders must be ruled out before proper treatment can be instituted.

Nerve root entrapment can only be relieved when the

Effects of Lumbar Hyperlordosis and Flexion on Spinal Nerve Roots

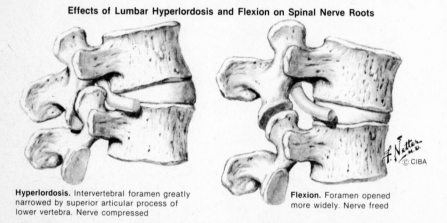

Hyperlordosis. Intervertebral foramen greatly narrowed by superior articular process of lower vertebra. Nerve compressed

Flexion. Foramen opened more widely. Nerve freed

Figure 4–2. The effects of lumbar swayback (hyperlordosis) and flexion on the spinal nerve roots. Notice how the nerves coming from the spine are pinched when the spine is placed in too much swayback, and how the nerve is decompressed when the spine is bent forward to open up the foramen. This is why it is so important to tuck the buttocks under the spine and pull your tummy in. (Copyright © 1980, CIBA Pharmaceutical Company)

patient bends forward in flexion, thus relieving the pinched nerves mechanically (Fig. 4–2). Usually the patient complains of severe nerve root pain when he is in an erect position, especially after prolonged walking or standing. The pain is generally relieved by sitting down and bending forward. Weight loss, abdominal exercises, and posture modification eliminate swayback and get the pelvis back underneath the spine, usually curing these patients (see Fig. 4–1).

Extrinsic Causes of Back Pain

Extrinsic causes of back pain (Fig. 4–1B) are also mechanical in origin, but are usually a result of conditions such as pelvic infections or uterine tumors in women. In men, extrinsic back pain is usually caused by inflammation or enlargement of the prostate gland. Pain from the gland is felt in the back (referred pain). The patient sees a doctor for relief of back pain, although this pain does not originate in the back.

Many conditions can cause extrinsic back pain; kidney stones, tumors, or a kidney infection can mimic low back pain, as well as hip disease, which is usually a result of arthritic changes and sends referred pain to the spine. Curvature of the spine (scoliosis) can cause secondary arthritic changes and extrinsic pain in adult life, especially if the curve is not treated in childhood or adolescence.

Most patients with scoliosis believe incorrectly that the spine will stop curving when they are mature. Nothing could be further from the truth: It has now been proven beyond a doubt that scoliosis will progress in most adults at the rate of 1 to 2 degrees per year and 5 to 8 degrees with each pregnancy. Women who have 25- or 30-degree curves at age nineteen or twenty can have 50- and 60-degree curves at age thirty-five or forty. Secondary arthritic changes occur in their spines, especially after several pregnancies. Eventually they have low back pain, associated with nerve-root entrapment problems and spinal stenosis. Most problems can be solved with exercise programs and weight loss; however, occasionally spinal surgery is necessary to relieve not only the nerve-root entrapment but also to correct the scoliosis as much as possible, depending on the patient's age.

Sacroiliac sprains are torn ligaments at the sacroiliac joint. There are right and left joints, one on each side of the spine where the sacrum joins the pelvic bone. Sometimes the ligaments holding the sacrum and the wing of the ilium (pelvic bone) together can be injured, or even be the source of infection.

Patients with sacroiliac sprains develop severe low back pain which can only be helped if diagnosed correctly. If an infection is present, it must be cleared up before the pain will subside. If there is a sprain as a result of some type of injury or inappropriate activity, the patient should be under a doctor's supervision and must rest before the pain will subside.

DEGENERATIVE DISORDERS

The most common degenerative disorders that affect the spine and cause back pain are *spondylosis, osteoarthritis, slipped or herniated discs,* and *spinal stenosis.* These will be discussed in order.

Spondylosis

Spondylosis is a condition caused by degenerative changes in the vertebral disc area (Fig. 4–3A). The disc itself is absorbed as a result of mechanical abuse in the disc area as well as repeated stresses and strains throughout life. A person who was a very active athlete as a youngster will often pay for his athletic prowess as he ages.

Spondylosis can cause a marked collapse in the lower lumbar spine and bone formation with spurring. These conditions lead to severe lumbar pain and restriction of motion. Everyone over the age of forty starts to develop some form of degenerative spondylosis and osteoarthritis (the combination of these conditions is called degenerative hypertrophic spondylitis), but these conditions, which can be likened to the rusting of a car, can be retarded if we take good care of our bodies, eat properly, take dietary supplements, and exercise daily.

Osteoarthritis

Osteoarthritis is a degenerative disorder that affects the major joints. In the spine the small facet joints at the back of the spine are affected (Fig. 4–3A). Osteoarthritis and spondylosis usually

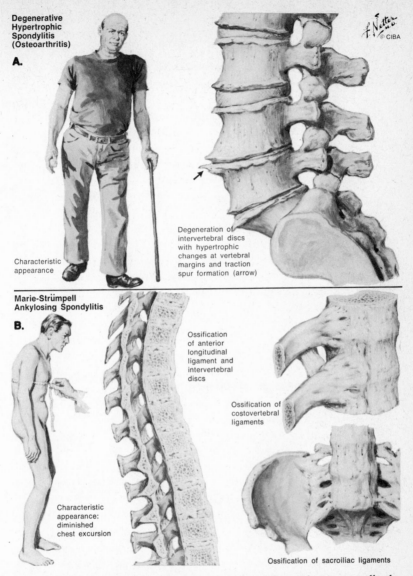

Degenerative Hypertrophic Spondylitis (Osteoarthritis)

A.

Characteristic appearance

Degeneration of intervertebral discs with hypertrophic changes at vertebral margins and traction spur formation (arrow)

Marie-Strümpell Ankylosing Spondylitis

B.

Ossification of anterior longitudinal ligament and intervertebral discs

Ossification of costovertebral ligaments

Characteristic appearance: diminished chest excursion

Ossification of sacroiliac ligaments

Figure 4–3. A. Degenerative hypertrophic spondylitis. This is actually the arthritis that forms in the joint made up of two vertebral bodies. It consists of degenerative changes which are the effect of mechanical abuse to the spine as well as the effect of aging. Patients can usually be markedly helped by weight reduction to relieve the loading on the vertebrae, and also by a proper exercise regimen to keep the joints mobile. B. Marie-Strümpell ankylosing spondylitis is a form of rheumatoid arthritis in males. It consists of bony formation in the ligaments and discs holding the vertebrae together and causes not only severe pain, but a progressive forward bending in the thoracic spine (kyphosis). (Copyright © 1980, CIBA Pharmaceutical Company)

occur together, affecting many major parts of the skeleton simultaneously. (The spondylitic changes occur at the disc level in front of the vertebral body, and the osteoarthritic changes occur in the facet joints in back). Osteoarthritis affects the knees, ankles, and hips just as frequently as it does the spine. It is part of the normal aging process. Osteoarthritis differs from rheumatoid arthritis in that it is *not* an inflammatory condition; the affected person does not have bouts of fever or inflammation.

Osteoarthritis is the most common form of arthritis and is typical of the aging process. Marked symptoms are rare before the age of fity, although joints that have been injured by fractures or other trauma in early adult life, either through an accident or repeated stresses such as athletic injuries, may be affected earlier. Osteoarthritis causes general breakdown of the cartilage of the joint; bony growths called spurs form around the edges of the joint (Fig. 4–3). When these spurs break free and float into the joint, especially in joints such as the knee or hip, we call them joint mice. Joint mice can float throughout the joint and cause the joint to lock and suddenly give way. In the spine joint mice are relatively uncommon. Disability is more likely to follow arthritic changes in the small facet joints in the posterior portion of the spine. This generally leads to significant pain and limitation of spinal motion. As the pain increases and bone formation continues, more severe conditions such as spinal stenosis occur.

Osteoarthritis usually occurs in people who are overweight and who have a genetic predisposition to this condition. If your ancestors were people who complained of arthritis with age, you are predisposed to the same problems as you age. The symptoms are particularly common in people who have engaged in years of heavy labor and are now underexercised.

The best treatment for all forms of arthritis is to stay slim and thus reduce the burden of weight on your joints. Plenty of rest, especially during an acute attack when the joint is swollen, is essential. As the attack subsides, the joint should be gently moved through its range of motion to preserve total mobility. Plenty of exercise is necessary to prevent muscle atrophy and joint stiffness. Your physician can usually tell you exactly which exercises are permissible. Sexual activity seems to be helpful in certain forms of arthritis, and psychologically is of great help also. Exercise, in most instances, should restore mobility and strength with the least possible amount of pain.

People with arthritis should maintain good posture and breathing habits and should use a firm mattress and try *warm* tub baths for fifteen to twenty minutes two or three times a day. Water for the tub baths should never be too hot, because people with arthritic changes are insensitive to temperature and may be severely burned. Occasionally ice packs alternated with hot compresses are extremely helpful, but should only be applied with the direction of a physical therapist. Regular massage and physiotherapy can also be very helpful to aid in relieving pain. Vitamins and mineral supplements that include calcium are always helpful, along with a warm, dry climate. In some cases, shoes with soft rubber heels or crepe soles will reduce jarring to the hips and spine. Strenuous work such as heavy lifting and straining should always be avoided, and occupations that require long periods of sitting or standing in one position are harmful. Corsets and braces should only be used to relieve acute bouts of pain.

Medications for Arthritis The tremendous number of drugs for arthritis, available either over the counter or through prescriptions, confuse the average person. Of all these drugs, the mainstay of treatment is *aspirin*. Doses as high as three or four aspirin tablets every four hours have been used successfully in patients with rheumatoid arthritis to reduce swelling and alleviate pain. However, aspirin can cause severe stomach upset and lead to ulcer formation, as well as to hearing damage and dizziness in some cases. Self-medication with large amounts of drugs should always be discouraged, and the help of a physician should be sought for severe arthritis. Hormone injections and steroid drugs should also be taken only under close supervision.

Approximately forty years ago, when *cortisone* and its derivatives were first introduced to the health-care field, we felt that the breakthrough would be fantastic for arthritic sufferers. However, serious side effects soon appeared. Although cortisone drugs can be of great help, they should only be used for short periods of time since prolonged use can cause marked bony absorption, as well as unsightly hair formation all over the body. Other side effects that are extremely dangerous include suppression of the adrenal glands. Cortisone is a very potent drug that should never be used without medical supervision.

Indomethacin (Indocin) is a relatively helpful drug and has been used during the last five years for various forms of osteoarthritis and rheumatoid arthritis. It must be given in proper doses, and because it can cause eye problems if used for a long period of time, the patient should be examined by an eye specialist every six months. It is dangerous in children, pregnant women, nursing mothers, and people with ulcers.

Phenylbutazone (Butazolidin) is a very common drug used not only in humans, but also in racehorses. It often relieves the symptoms of pain, but also has side effects when taken for long periods. These include irritation of the stomach, water retention, and stomach ulcers. Phenylbutazone can also depress the normal blood count and should not be taken with blood-thinning drugs such as Coumadin, especially in patients with heart disease.

Many other medications such as folic acid, zinc sulfate, gold pills, and hormonal therapy with agents such as the prostaglandins are also available. Most have not been proven to be as helpful as the basic aspirin-type drugs over the long run. Again, most of these drugs should only be taken with medical supervision. Medical specialists, known as rheumatologists, have spent their lives studying these conditions and are best qualified to provide long-term supervision and immediate help during acute flare-ups.

In recent years a drug called *dimethyl sulfoxide (DMSO)* has been shown to reduce pain and help improve joint motion in people with all forms of arthritis. It is a by-product of the wood pulp industry, and for many years was discarded until it was found to be absorbed quickly through the skin and directly into the bloodstream. It has proved to be tremendously effective in athletes, in people with joint swelling and pain, and in the treatment of animals. However, it also appears to cause cataracts in the eye and is still under intense clinical investigation. Although it is available in some areas of this country and in Canada, the facts on DMSO are not all in, and it should only be used under the strictest medical supervision.

The Slipped or Herniated Disc (Nucleus Pulposus)

The term *slipped disc* has been used by both medical and nonmedical people for the last fifty years. Actually the word *slip* is misleading, since the disc is located between two vertebral bodies and does not in any way slip. Instead, degenerative changes occur in the disc material itself, especially in the central nucleus pulposus, which is surrounded by the tough fibrous anulus, that encases each disc. When degenerative changes occur in the disc, the nucleus pulposus tends to squeeze out, usually through the weakest area of the anulus, which happens to be *at the rear of the disc*. The squeezing action resembles putty squirting out of a putty gun. Since the disc material squeezes out into the spinal canal, it usually pinches nerve roots against the bony elements that make up the roof of the spinal canal (see Figs. 4-4A and B).

Although herniated discs usually follow an injury in a person with poor muscle tone who suddenly lifts a lawn mower or tries to open a stuck garage door, they can also occur in young people. In my own practice, I have had to surgically correct herniated discs in many children under the age of eighteen who had very severe nerve pressure caused by the disc pressing directly on either the fourth, fifth lumbar, or first sacral nerve root. Why does a degenerative type of disc disease affect some young people? We suspect that these children are victims of a poorly understood condition called an autoimmune disease. This type of disease causes us to become allergic to certain cells in our own body, and our body tends to actually reject these elements inside it and cause degenerative breakdown. Autoimmune disease is evidently the cause of disc disease in young children, since sometimes histories of serious injury are not present. Whatever the cause, disc disease in 90 percent of all cases involves the lowest two lumbar vertebrae, and disc rupture and herniation occurs between the fourth and fifth lumbar vertebrae or between the fifth lumbar vertebra and the sacrum.

Usually the patient with a herniated disc has specific symptoms and a history of severe pain down the back and outer part of the thigh and calf, sometimes accompanied by shooting pain to the foot. A well-trained medical examiner can usually make the diagnosis without much difficulty in a classic case. However, in cases where the history or physical findings are not altogether clear, the diagnostic abilities of the finest physician can be taxed.

The physical examination will often show changes in the reflexes, usually at the ankle or knee, and muscle wasting, such as atrophy of the calf or thigh muscles on the affected side. Straight leg raising—a test in which the leg is straightened with the patient lying on the back, then raised to form a 90-degree

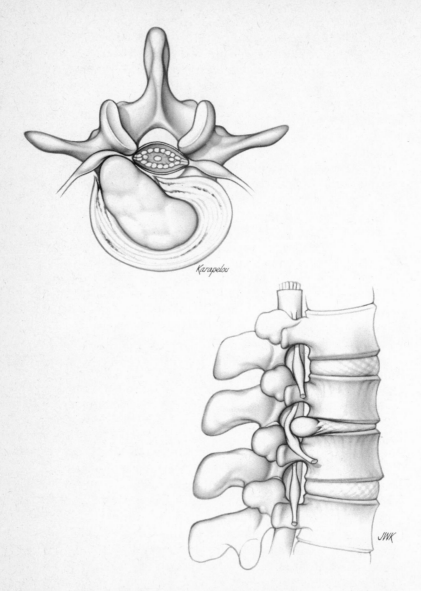

Figure 4–4. A. This diagram illustrates a herniated disc pressing directly on the nerve as it exits from the lumbar spinal canal. The central nucleus pulposus squeezes out like putty from a putty gun and presses on the nerve, causing intense pain in the lower back which often radiates down the back of the leg. B. A side view, showing the ruptured or herniated disc pressing on the nerve root as it makes its exit from the lumbar spine. (© Columbia University 1981)

angle with the spine—is almost impossible for patients with a herniated disc. In addition, herniated discs often cause loss of sensation in portions of the lower extremities. All of these findings together will usually help an astute physician make the diagnosis (Fig. 4-5).

HERNIATED NUCLEUS PULPOSUS (LUMBAR); CLINICAL FEATURES

LEVEL OF HERNIATION	PAIN	NUMBNESS	WEAKNESS	ATROPHY	REFLEXES
4th L — L3-4 DISC; 4th L NERVE ROOT	Lower Back, Hip Postero-Lateral Thigh, Anterior Leg	Anteromedial Thigh, Knee	Quadriceps	Quadriceps	Diminished Knee Jerk
5th L — L4-5 DISC; 5th L NERVE ROOT	Over Sacro-Iliac Joint, Hip, Lateral Thigh, and Leg	Lateral Leg, Web of Great Toe	Weakness of Dorsiflexion of Great Toe and Foot; Difficulty Walking on Heels; Foot Drop May Occur	Minor	Changes Uncommon (Absent or Diminished Post. Tibial Reflex)
1st S — L5-S1 DISC; 1st S NERVE ROOT	Over Sacro-Iliac Joint, Hip, Postero-Lateral and Leg To Heel	Back of Calf; Lateral Heel, Foot, and Toe	May Affect Plantar Flexion Great Toe; of Foot and Difficulty Walking on Toes	Gastrocnemius and Soleus	Diminished or Absent Ankle Jerk
5th L — MASSIVE MIDLINE PROTRUSION S1-5	Lower Back, Thighs, Legs, and/or Perineum Depending on Level of Lesion; May be Bilateral	Variable; Thighs, Legs, Feet, and/or Perineum; May be Bilateral	Variable Paralysis or Paresis of Legs and/or Bowel, and Bladder Incontinence	May be Extensive	Diminished or Absent Ankle Jerk

Figure 4–5. This chart illustrates the usual pain pattern and findings that the doctor uses to diagnose the level of a disc herniation in the lumbar spine. By referring to the chart, one can see that pressure on different nerves of the lumbar area can cause different groups of symptoms and pain. By the use of proper diagnostic methods, the exact location of the disc protrusion can be located and adequately treated. (Adapted from original artwork by Frank H. Netter, M.D., from Clinical Symposia, Copyright © 1980, CIBA Pharmaceutical Company.)

Approximately 85 percent of all people who have a single episode of disc herniation can be well treated with absolute bed rest and the use of muscle relaxants and anti-inflammatory drugs; sometimes the bed rest must continue for at least four to six weeks. Most patients who have a single episode of disc herniation can learn to lead a perfectly normal life and eventually go back to full activity if they do what is necessary to prevent further problems. Often, however, patients burn the candle at both ends, and disc disease becomes recurrent, with increasing disability. If herniation recurs, further examination in the hospital is necessary. A myelogram and a computer tomogram (CT scan) along with other diagnostic tests to be discussed later will help clinch the diagnosis. Even recurrent herniations usually do not require surgery and can be treated with various forms of traction and manipulation. Surgery should generally be a last resort for people with herniated disc disease unless there is progressive nerve injury and muscle weakness in the lower extremities.

Disc herniation can also occur in the neck (the cervical spine) and cause the same type of symptoms in our arms and hands as it does in the legs. In these cases, the same diagnostic tests can be used to delineate the presence of a herniated disc and to determine what level it is at (Fig. 4-6). Nonoperative treatment can be of help in 90 percent of cases. In rare cases the pinched nerve must be decompressed and the bones fused together so as to prevent further disc-space collapse and recurrence of symptoms.

Herniated discs can be prevented in the same way that all other conditions affecting the spine are avoided. People who are soft, poorly muscled, overweight, and underexercised are sitting ducks for herniated disc disease, especially if they have inherited a predisposition. Keeping your body weight normal, paying constant attention to proper diet, and exercising to keep the cells and muscles of your body in their best possible condition is the finest form of prevention.

Spinal Stenosis—Nerve Root Entrapment Syndrome or Pinched Nerves

When I was a medical student, my father was in his early seventies. He constantly complained to me of pain, numbness,

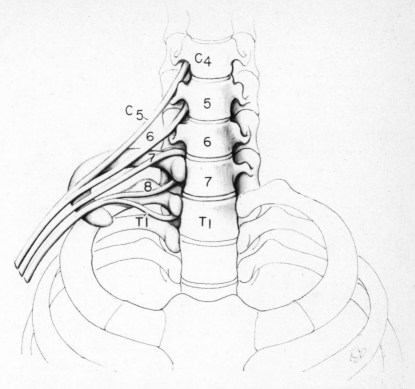

Figure 4–6. The nerves of the lower part of the neck make up the brachial plexus. This consists of the nerves of the fifth, sixth, seventh, and eighth cervical roots, as well as the first thoracic nerve root. Sometimes patients can have an extra or accessory rib in the neck which can cause direct pressure on the nerves forming the brachial plexus and lead to severe pain in the neck and arm. Herniated discs affecting any one of these levels can also mimic the same symptoms.

and tingling in his legs, especially during the night. He always awakened at three or four in the morning with the feeling that his legs were falling asleep. The only relief was to get out of bed and walk around the house for an hour or two. Crouching in a forward position would often produce an immediate return of sensation to his legs and toes. I misdiagnosed his ailment as a circulatory condition and sent him to a vascular specialist who examined the arteries of his pelvis and lower extremities. Naturally, by the age of seventy, all of us have some hardening of the arteries, and we dismiss many symptoms as related to

Pathology of Spinal Stenosis

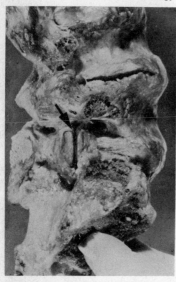

A. Protuberant osteophytes on both facets of lateral spinal articulation

B. Circumferential and radial tears of anulus fibrosus lead to nucleus pulposus herniation

Inferior articular process of superior vertebra

Superior articular process of inferior vertebra

C. Central spinal canal narrowed by enlargement of inferior articular processes of superior vertebra. Lateral recesses narrowed by subluxation and osteophytic enlargement of superior articular processes of inferior vertebra

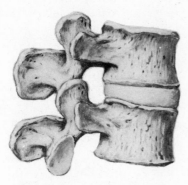 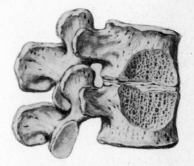

D. Properly spaced lumbar vertebrae with normal intervertebral disc

E. Vertebrae approximated as a result of loss of disc height. Superior articular process of lower vertebra has encroached on foramen. Cutaway reveals internal disruption of disc

Figure 4–7. Spinal stenosis and the effects of disc degeneration and bony overgrowth of the facet joints on narrowing the spinal canal. Notice how the bony spurs growing from the facet joints narrow down the canal through which the spinal nerves can pass and make their exit to the lower extremities. In addition, Figures D and E show what happens when the disc between two of the vertebrae degenerates and narrows. The little foramen tends to narrow because the disc itself is absorbed and causes pressure directly on the nerve roots exiting from the lumbar spine. (Copyright © 1980, CIBA Pharmaceutical Company)

circulatory disorders. At that time in my medical career—and in fact until just recently—no one knew of a group of spinal disorders caused by spinal stenosis, the disease my father had.

Spinal stenosis is a degenerative disease caused by spondylosis in the intervertebral disc and osteoarthritis of the facet joints in the lumbar spine. Little bony spurs form around the small facet joints at the posterior portion of the spine, causing them to encroach into the spinal canal itself. The enlarged joints narrow the canal and prevent the nerves from exiting from the spine. In many cases the nerves are actually compressed by the bony overgrowths, causing a nerve root entrapment syndrome. My father had this condition; when he bent his spine forward and squatted he temporarily eliminated the swayback posture that caused the bony spurs to press on his spinal nerves and relieved the pressure by opening up the spinal spaces (see Figs. 1–3 and 4–7).

In addition to the hypertrophy of the facet joints in the back of the spinal vertebrae, the disc is also affected. With degenerative changes the disc volume decreases, causing the size of the little window (or foramen) through which the nerve roots exit to decrease as well. The nerve root is then so severely kinked that the entire spinal canal becomes narrowed. The narrowed canal compresses the spinal nerves like a rubber band would if it were wrapped tightly around the finger (Figs. 4–7D and E).

Spinal stenosis can cause marked pain and severe disability in the back and lower extremities. It is an extremely common condition in aging adults and is probably present in almost everyone over the age of seventy to some degree. A previous injury such as a fall, with fracture of a vertebra, will increase the chances of getting spinal stenosis; people who have a history of arthritis in their family are also genetically predisposed to this condition. It is only in the last five years that spinal stenosis has really become known among physicians throughout the world. In a monograph published by the CIBA Pharmaceutical Company in December of 1980, the condition is very well outlined. (This monograph, "Low Back Pain," can be obtained from CIBA-GEIGY Corporation, Summit, New Jersey 07901. The cost is two dollars per copy.)

The diagnosis of spinal stenosis is very complicated because patients have such bizarre complaints and symptoms. I am convinced that in the past, patients with stenosis were often listened to politely and dismissed because very few physical findings were detected on examination to account for their symptoms. Patients can have reflexes that are completely normal, normal muscle power, and a normal range of motion in the lower extremities and still have marked spinal stenosis (just as my father did). Now that excellent X-ray techniques such as computerized tomography (CT scanning) are available, we can diagnose this condition with great accuracy, usually on an outpatient basis. In fact, the ability to image with various types of X rays and bone scans is a tremendous diagnostic advantage, and these techniques are being improved almost on a daily basis. We can now get a computerized scan of the entire spinal canal in multiple planes, so that we can not only look inside the spinal canal, but also completely around it without in any way hurting or invading your body.

The best treatment for mild cases of spinal stenosis is posture training to get rid of excessive lumbar lordosis or swayback, weight reduction, and muscle exercises to improve muscle tone. In approximately 80 percent of patients, spinal stenosis can be relieved in this way; but in certain patients with progressive nerve changes, surgery is indicted and decompression of the spinal nerves can be done very successfully by a skilled surgeon (see Chapters 8 and 9).

TRAUMA

Trauma is a word usually associated with injury. The injury can be extremely mild, such as a strain or a sprain, or it can be something severe such as an actual fracture of a bone.

Lumbar Strain

Strains of muscles are actually small tears within the muscles themselves, whereas a *sprain* is usually an injury to a ligament that holds bone to bone. It is possible to have sprains in the spine, but they are more common around other major weight-bearing joints such as the ankle or the knee. However, muscle strains—which are either acute or chronic—occur with great frequency. An *acute strain* is usually one that comes on rather suddenly; the best example is the strain suffered by the so-called weekend athlete. Many of us are rather sedentary during the week and either sit behind a desk or have some other static job where not too much energy or muscular activity is expended. Then suddenly Saturday comes, and if it happens to be a beautiful day, we think nothing of going out and playing six sets of tennis after one or two weeks of no activity at all! This results in what I call the *weekend athlete syndrome*, a syndrome of frequent muscular injuries, especially around the spine. On Monday mornings five or six patients generally call my office. They are in severe pain and want to be seen that morning. Usually they have participated in some ill-advised activity, with strenuous frenzy, over the weekend. Another weekend athlete is the father who is trying to show his twelve-year-old Little Leaguer how he used to slide into second base ("when he himself was a baseball star"). Little League fathers are extremely common and show up in our emergency room frequently, especially during the spring when the baseball season is about to start, and in the fall when the football season is underway. Many of us do not realize that our muscles have changed with the years, and that the fine physiques we had when we were in our teens and early twenties are no longer present! Trying to demonstrate how we used to return a football punt ninety-five yards, while eluding swarms of downfield tacklers, will usually result in a week of bed rest with a heating pad and a prescription for muscle relaxants.

Chronic lumbar strain is usually the result of repeated acute strains. You've probably heard about people who have sprained their ankles repeatedly over a period of years. Finally, the ankle is so weak that it sprains with the slightest provocation, and they have difficulty walking at all. The same thing can happen in the lumbar spine, and strains become so common and chronic that people are afraid to do practically anything. *The worst thing about having severe lumbar muscle spasm is the fear that it is going to happen again!* It is like waiting for the other shoe to drop. If you have injured yourself during gardening or some other pursuit, you will be frightened to try those pursuits again for fear of reactivating the original injury. Usually chronic lumbar strains can be handled extremely well by doing the PRE exercises outlined in Chapter 3. The six PREs, done *daily* once you have back pain, along with the five KPEs, will do more to help your back and prevent chronic lumbar strain than any other treatment!

Compression Fractures

Fracture of the Vertebral Body Compression fractures are actually injuries to vertebrae which collapse in a wedge shape, much like a compressed styrofoam block (Fig. 4–8). Compression fractures usually affect the bodies of the vertebrae themselves and are the result of bone weakening with loss of bone content. Loss of content is seen in osteoporosis, where the amount of bone inside the vertebral body itself is diminished, weakening the vertebra substantially. Unfortunately, compression fractures also occur very frequently after tumors have invaded the vertebrae.

Sometimes a patient is admitted to the hospital with multiple compression fractures following a fall. By examining small portions of bone through the method of a biopsy, we can determine if the fracture is a result of weakness of the bone (osteoporosis) or of a tumor. Compression fractures usually occur in people who are over the age of sixty when the bones have been weakened by osteoporosis. Even a relatively slight fall, such as falling down the steps or slipping on the ice, can cause multiple compression fractures in weakened vertebrae; the fractures are most common in the lower thoracic or upper lumbar vertebrae. In most cases a brace or corset is used for several months, and the results are quite good; surgery is rarely necessary. With a proper diet, bone minerals are increased, and patients end up with relatively stable spinal conditions with a minimum of pain.

Fractures of Transverse Processes The transverse processes are small handles that protrude from each side of the lumbar vertebrae and form an area for muscle attachment (Fig. 1–3). Sometimes with extremely severe muscle pull and spasm, as would be seen in an auto accident, the transverse process can actually be torn from the side of the vertebrae and become a loose fragment. Fractures almost always heal very well and rarely cause serious problems. The important thing is to make the diagnosis. These fractures usually cause severe pain and muscle spasm because of bleeding inside the area where the fracture occurs. Usually more than one transverse process is ripped free. The patient must stay in bed for one or two weeks, until the pain and muscle spasm have subsided.

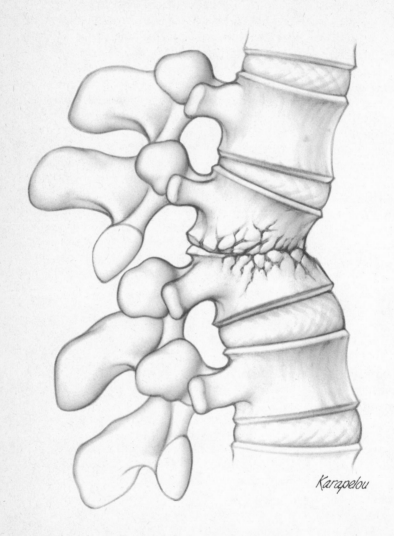

Figure 4–8. This diagram illustrates a compression fracture of an upper lumbar vertebra. Notice how the vertebral bodies collapse, causing not only destruction of the bodies themselves, but separation of the facet joints behind them. Mild compression fractures usually heal without incidence after four to eight weeks. More severe fractures sometimes require surgical stabilization and decompression if nerve roots have been injured. (© Columbia University 1981)

Seat-Belt Injuries Auto accidents are increasing throughout the world. In fact, one out of every two drivers will be involved in a serious auto accident during his or her driving career. However, in a study done in Sweden, *all* drivers who wore lap and shoulder belts survived collisions taking place under sixty miles per hour. There is no question that seat belts are extremely valuable; they have certainly saved many thousands of lives and prevented numerous injuries. Seat belts restrain a person directly at the waist when a vehicle is involved in a direct deceleration accident, such as in hitting a tree or another vehicle. In this type of accident, the victim's upper trunk slides forward while the seat belt holds the lower trunk in place. This motion can easily result in a severe vertebral fracture and also often causes injuries to the spinal cord and the nerve roots. However, I would like to point out again that had the patient not worn the seat belt, he would probably have been killed by an accident of that severity. In general, seat belts are an extremely safe and important preventive device and should always be worn. When newer, improved restraint devices such as the air-bag system are perfected, spinal injuries caused by low- and high-speed accidents should decrease significantly.

Subluxated Facet Joints (Facet Syndrome)

In the lumbar spine there are basically three joints. The large, broad joint that is on a parallel plane with the ground is the joint formed by the two vertebral bodies, held apart by the disc (which acts as a shock absorber). In addition, there are two small joints, one on each side in the back, which are called facet joints (Fig. 1–3). These are actually small joints that have the same linings and cartilage as our knee and ankle joints. Although these joints are held together with a very strong system of ligaments, they can sometimes slip out of place and dislocate. When the dislocation is not complete we call it a subluxation. Subluxation can be extremely serious and painful. The facet joints are probably subluxated when a person complains that he cannot move or straighten up at all after a minor injury. Lifting a lawn mower into the back of a car, or moving a heavy piece of furniture like a piano can cause such an injury.

Facet syndrome is probably the ailment which chiropractors and osteopaths are able to treat most successfully;

remarkable cures are sometimes obtained through manipulatory techniques. A spinal adjustment at the hands of an expert in this technique can be extremely effective.

Spondylolysis and Spondylolisthesis

These very long and complicated terms are derived from Greek words which mean *to slip*. For some reason that we do not yet understand, certain of the lower lumbar vertebrae—usually the fifth lumbar vertebra, and in some instances the fourth—become weak. The weakness occurs in the area called the neck or isthmus of the vertebra. With prolonged stress, the area cracks, and the back section of the vertebra tends to separate from the vertebral body (Fig. 4–9). This condition is called *spondylolysis*. Occasionally the affected vertebral body actually slides forward on the body below it. The condition is then called *spondylolisthesis;* the degree of severity is indicated as Grade I, II, III, and IV, depending on how far forward the vertebra has slipped. In a Grade IV slip, the vertebra has slid completely forward on the body below it. Of course if this happens, the spinal nerves are stretched and kinked, causing severe pain, especially down the back of the legs. Patients also have marked spasm of the hamstring muscles, which prevents bending forward at the waist with the knees straight.

We do not completely understand the causes of spondylolysis or spondylolisthesis, although we do know that they have some genetic basis. Usually if one of the parents had either one of these conditions, a certain number of the offspring have them too. The two conditions are seen in approximately 5 percent of the world population and, in my own practice, I see many families in which two or three members have exactly the same condition. What we do know is that spondylolisthesis is basically a stress fracture that is genetically predisposed. In other words, a patient must first have a genetic weakness, and then repeated stresses such as gymnastics, ballet dancing, or tackle football may cause the weakened area to finally fracture and separate. I have never seen a patient younger than the age of five with spondylolisthesis; usually it occurs in the teenage years, especially in children subjected to repeated shearing stresses such as occur in contact sports.

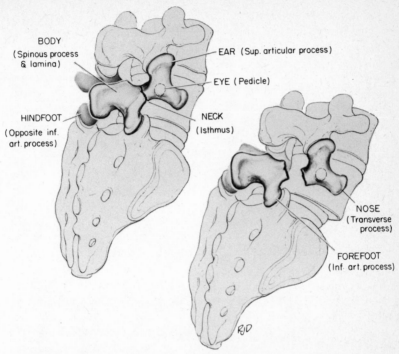

BODY
(Spinous process
& lamina)

EAR (Sup. articular process)

EYE (Pedicle)

HINDFOOT
(Opposite inf.
art. process)

NECK
(Isthmus)

NOSE
(Transverse
process)

FOREFOOT
(Inf. art. process)

Figure 4–9. Spondylolysis and spondylolisthesis. These long Greek words describe a slippage that occurs usually in the lumbar spine, where the posterior element of the vertebrae develops a stress fracture that is genetically predisposed and allows the body of the vertebra to slide forward on the vertebra below it.

In many cases spondylolysis and spondylolisthesis cause only occasional aches and pains. The patient can learn to live with the condition as long as he is X-rayed every year or two to see that further slippage doesn't occur. However, sometimes the pain and hamstring muscle spasm become so severe that surgery is required. The affected area is decompressed by removing the loose elements to the rear of the vertebral body and freeing up the nerve roots where they are kinked and compressed. A spinal fusion is usually necessary to weld the lower two vertebrae to the sacrum. In the hands of highly skilled orthopaedic surgeons, the results are usually very satisfactory; almost all patients can go back to a completely normal life.

METABOLIC DISORDERS

Osteoporosis

Osteoporosis is the most common disease of bones encountered in my clinical practice. In this condition, bone becomes less dense and the amount of bone in the body—that is, the total bony mass—decreases. Most men and women, after the age of forty, start to lose bone mineral, but in postmenopausal women the decrease can be extremely severe. Although osteoporosis can occur in children and young adults, it is rare in the young population. It is most common in women; three out of four are affected to some degree after menopause. Interestingly, women who weigh less than 120 pounds and are of average height develop osteoporosis at almost twice the rate of women who are heavier than 140 pounds. The medical reasons for this are not clear.

Osteoporosis can be caused by a calcium deficiency in the diet, either because we are not ingesting enough calcium or because calcium is not being absorbed properly. It can also occur following long treatment with cortisone-type drugs and can be made worse by immobilizing the skeleton, especially after injury. A leg that has been in a cast or in traction for many months will be withered and atrophied compared to the other leg when the treatment is finished. An X ray taken of the immobilized bones will show much less bone mineral than on the normal side. Also, bone on the treated side will be extremely weak as a result of osteoporosis caused by immobilization. Weakness and atrophy can be improved by active physical therapy and proper diet.

In women with osteoporosis, back pain becomes chronic and very disabling. Usually the onset of pain is slow and insidious, beginning at the age of forty to fifty. In most women osteoporosis affects all the bones of the skeleton. Certainly it is a major factor in hip fractures, and we now know that women in their eighties and nineties actually break their hip first, sometimes with the slightest stress, and then fall down as a result of the fracture. These women usually have marked osteoporosis.

Persistent pain in the thoracic spine is usually the major symptom of osteoporosis in women over forty-five or fifty. If the patient also has a fall, the osteoporotic spine can suffer multiple compression fractures and make the situation much worse. Unfortunately, by the time osteoporosis is first seen on X ray, 30 percent to 50 percent of the bone in the vertebrae has already been lost.

Proper Diet for Osteoporosis

What can be done for osteoporosis? Basically, a diet that includes calcium supplements or bone meal and high levels of calcium (found in milk and cheese) is very helpful. Vitamin D supplements should also be taken to insure proper absorption of calcium by the intestines. Vitamin D and calcium should not be taken in large amounts, to avoid vitamin D poisoning. These diets, along with fluoride intake, should only be undertaken in consultation with a physician well trained in the treatment of metabolic diseases.

Occasionally estrogen shots are given to help delay the menopause and make this transition smoother for women; however, administration of female hormones (such as estrogen), unless extremely carefully regulated, can cause an increase in osteoporosis and breast tumors. Estrogen in itself does not rebuild bone that has been lost, but can prevent further bone loss in some women. It can also relieve pain and cause an increased sense of well-being. Estrogen should only be taken in regulated doses at specific times of the month, and only under the strictest medical supervision.

Generally, the best way to avoid osteoporosis is to eat a balanced diet that includes calcium supplements as well as vitamin D, and follow a daily exercise program. Swimming and walking are especially helpful. We know for sure that leading an active life with plenty of regular exercise is the best way to prevent osteoporosis. Never let yourself become totally immobilized; the worst thing an elderly person can do is retreat to a rocking chair or become a total shut-in. Men and women of advanced years often become recluses after losing their mates, and no longer eat properly. They then develop severe vitamin deficiencies, and because they don't eat enough milk products— such as ice cream or cheese—they become extremely deficient in minerals. Many elderly adults are on some form of diet and cut back on milk and dairy products because of their high caloric values, thus depriving their bodies of the much-needed minerals required for daily bone metabolism.

Calcium supplements are seldom necessary in early life because calcium conservation in growing children is very efficient. It is not just the calcium levels in our bodies that are important, but the calcium-phosphorous ratio in our diets as well. If the phosphorous level is too high in relation to the calcium, the bones tend to be absorbed. What must be preserved is the proper relationship. The average American gets only about half as much calcium as he really needs. Carbonated soft drinks contain a great amount of phosphorous; if too many of these drinks are taken, an imbalance in the calcium-phosphorous ratio will result, leading to bone reabsorption.

The whole secret to minimizing osteoporosis is *prevention*. An active, healthy person who eats a properly supplemented diet should live well into his or her eighties or nineties without difficulty, as long as the pursuit of life is vigorous and laced with the proper amounts of exercise and dietary supplements. I belong to the New York Athletic Club and am impressed with the many octogenarians I see there who participate in very strenuous activities, such as handball and water polo. These people are in extremely sound physical condition; some who are in their eighties can do as many as seventy-five to one hundred pushups. These people have been physically active for fifty or sixty years and have never let a day go by without eating properly and taking vitamin and mineral supplements. Their good health is testimony to the importance of taking care of the body you have been given. We are only issued one body to last our entire life. Although we can replace portions of it with reasonable substitutes, we still must maintain the integrity of our bones, muscles, and ligaments with proper diet and exercise if we want to have healthy and happy golden years.

Osteoporosis should not be confused with *osteomalacia*, another disorder in which a disturbance of calcium metabolism causes a decrease in the density of the skeleton. Osteomalacia in adults is similar to rickets in children, and is the result of a vitamin D deficiency. Fortunately, in this country osteomalacia is rare; it is only seen in people from extremely depressed socioeconomic areas where diets are still totally inadequate.

A word of caution about dietary supplements. As people become more health-conscious and rely more on health foods, we must be careful not to harm ourselves. A recent study of dolomite (a rock containing calcium and magnesium), which is becoming a favorite dietary supplement, has shown that it also contains toxic minerals such as lead, arsenic, mercury, and aluminum. Dr. H. J. Roberts, of the Palm Beach Institute for Medical Research in Florida, has shown unexpected high doses of these elements in patients ingesting considerable amounts of dolomite. Be wary of taking supplements and drugs that are not medically proven to be of help to your body. Also, avoid the American mania that if one megavitamin is good for you, massive doses will be even better. Severe toxicity can result in cataracts, kidney stones, hearing loss, and other yet unknown dangerous side effects.

INFECTIONS

Acute Infections of the Spine

Infections of the spine, fortunately, are extremely rare. They may be either acute (of a short and severe course) or chronic. Infections of the spine are usually systemic. The term *systemic* means that the bacterium goes through the bloodstream in some way, and sets up shop in and around the spine. Usually, because of the rich blood supply in the vertebral bodies, most infections occur directly inside a vertebra. However, in some cases the disc space itself can become infected.

Disc-space infections are usually acute and are occasionally found in children. Usually the patient has an extremely high fever and the diagnosis can be most difficult to make, even with an open biopsy. In an open biopsy, tissue is taken from the affected area and cultured so that any bacteria present will grow. Often, however, the bacteria do not grow, and the diagnosis is clouded and difficult to prove. These infections are usually carried by the blood to the spine from a primary source elsewhere in the body, such as the lungs or the genitourinary tract. In young patients, disc infections usually originate in the respiratory tract and are caused by staphylococcus bacteria. In older patients, the genitourinary tract is often the source of the original infection. In adult patients who have had a urologic procedure, the causative bacterium is almost always a gram-negative bacillus.

Disc-space infections in adults are usually associated with extremely severe low back pain, and can also develop one to eight weeks after spinal surgery involving an intervertebral disc. Disc-space infections may show absolutely no local signs other than pain, and occasionally even the patient's temperature is normal. The only abnormal laboratory finding is an elevated blood sedimentation rate, but the white blood count can be normal. As a rule, the best form of treatment for patients with disc-space infection is to place them on antibiotics, which are given on what we call an empirical basis because blood and wound cultures are frequently negative. Along with antibiotics, we immobilize patients from four to six months in a body cast to totally put their spines at rest, and the infection often comes under control.

Postoperative surgical infections can occur directly after an operation if enough bacteria enter the wound. Almost all surgical wounds are contaminated to a certain extent by bacteria because bacteria are present in the bloodstream and practically everywhere in and around the home, the body, and also in hospitals. However, most people who have surgical operations do not get infections because they have a certain resistance to bacteria. People who are in poor general health and are debilitated generally tend to get infections at a much greater rate than those who are in good health and whose bodies are properly nourished. Patients with postoperative wound infections usually have a localized abscess. However, if an overwhelming blood-borne infection develops, it can contribute to the development of severe spinal problems that can actually threaten the patient's life.

Chronic Infections of the Spine

In the past, most chronic infections of the spine causing severe disabling low back pain were a result of diseases like tuberculosis or osteomyelitis. The latter is a serious bone infection that usually involves the vertebrae, but may affect the other bones of the skeleton as well. Osteomyelitis is becoming more common, especially in areas where narcotic drug addiction is a problem. Many addicts inject their drugs with dirty needles and syringes and in filthy surroundings, which can lead to acute infections. The infection generally travels through the bloodstream and settles in the spine, leading to severe osteomyelitis of the vertebrae. Often the bacteria that cause these infections are extremely difficult to control. It is not uncommon for several addicts to use the same needle, thus transmitting not only the bacteria that cause osteomyelitis, but other organisms—such as those that cause syphilis—as well.

Tuberculosis of the spine is still a major cause of back pain, especially in underdeveloped countries. Moreover, because of crowded conditions in large cities in this country, the incidence of tuberculosis is rising again. People have developed a false sense of security about tuberculosis and feel that the problem has been solved in recent years. However, TB is certainly on the upswing; in our spine clinic at the Columbia-Presbyterian Medical Center, more cases have been diagnosed in the past year than we have seen in the last five years. The rise in tuberculosis is not only a result of people's lack of concern and failure to get proper tuberculin screening tests, but also of the increasing number of drug addicts and of people who live in sexually active communal groups where major diseases such as venereal diseases and tuberculosis are often transmitted at the same time.

Tuberculosis generally starts in the bony area of the vertebral body, causing a marked inflammatory reaction that results in severe loss of bone content and osteoporosis. The vertebral body yields easily to the compressive forces of the infection, and in many instances can collapse, causing a severe forward angulation of the spine that leads to an increase in kyphosis (hunchback). The infection can advance, destroying bones and eventually the intervertebral disc and adjacent vertebra. When several vertebrae collapse, the spinal cord may become compressed, paralyzing the patient. Abscesses can form and separate adjoining tissues from the spine. Some actually extend to the groin, where they spontaneously drain.

The patient with tubercular infection of the spine has severe back pain, weakness, loss of appetite, weight loss, nighttime sweating, and afternoon fever. Fortunately, treatment is extremely effective. Antibiotics are usually given in the form of three or four simultaneously administered medications. In some instances the abscess must be surgically drained and a spinal fusion done both in front and in back of the spine if the spinal cord shows evidence of compression and nerve damage.

CIRCULATORY DISORDERS

Abdominal Aortic Aneurysm

Circulatory disorders can cause back pain, especially in adult males. Now that people live longer, they are more prone to circulatory disorders. In males especially, the aorta (the largest blood vessel in the body, which rests directly in front of the vertebrae) can develop a weakness in its wall and bulge out, much like a weakened auto tire. The bulging is called an aneurysm. The aneurysm can cause very severe back pain because it wears away at the bodies of the vertebrae as it pulsates, causing bony weakness of the spine and invading the spinal column itself. The back pain closely mimics the pain caused by a herniated disc or a tumor. Prompt and accurate diagnosis is extremely important since a potentially fatal aneurysm rupture can occur.

Generally, the patients are males over fifty years of age who complain of severe, boring, and deep pain in the lumbar or pelvic region. The patient usually has evidence of arteriosclerosis (hardening of the arteries), and often complains of cold feet, numbness, and tingling. The patient may have had several undiagnosed small strokes in the past. During the physical examination, the doctor will find decreased pulses in the ankles and in back of the knees, as well as a decreased skin temperature in the lower extremities. The physician will feel a pulsating mass in the abdomen when he places his fingers directly over the bulge in the aorta and may hear a hissing sound through a stethoscope placed over the groin region. When the diagnosis is made promptly, the patient's life can be saved and his symptoms relieved.

Arteriosclerosis

Arteriosclerosis is commonly referred to as hardening of the arteries; it is caused by calcification of the blood vessels. Often it can lead to severe back pain by causing complete obstruction of the blood vessels going down one lower extremity. The symptoms can mimic those caused by a herniated disc or spinal cord tumor, and very accurate diagnosis is essential. The patient usually notices prolonged weakness after brief periods of walking and experiences pain occurring in the back, buttocks, thighs, and legs. He also notices fatigue, weakness, and atrophy (wasting away of the muscles), especially in the lower extremities. A man may become less potent sexually and complain of numbness and tingling of the lower extremities (Leriche's syndrome). The pulses in the lower extremities become weak and may even be absent on one side. Proper diagnosis with modern techniques usually allows superb corrections, with prompt and lasting relief. Often this condition is confused with spinal stenosis.

INFLAMMATORY DISORDERS

Rheumatoid Arthritis

The term *inflammatory disorders* refers to an entire group of arthritic conditions which can become extremely crippling and disabling. The group includes too many disorders to discuss each individually. *Rheumatoid arthritis* is the most important. Rheumatoid arthritis occurs in affected individuals at a very young age, usually between twenty and thirty-five. It is most common in women. The disease process affects the connective tissue of the bones and is seen in the hips, spine, and especially in the hands and feet. It usually begins with swelling and congestion of the finger and toe joints, with muscle pain and stiffness. Numbness and tingling of the hands and feet associated with fatigue and weight loss are most common. As the disease progresses, the wrists, elbows, knees, shoulders, hips, and spine become severely disabled, and the joints are actually destroyed. Most rheumatic diseases are autoimmune disorders. These disorders are not specifically understood at this time, but a great amount of research is being done throughout the world to uncover the exact causes of these conditions and to try to retard and prevent them completely.

Women with rheumatoid arthritis usually have episodes of very severe symptoms interspersed with periods of marked remission (where the condition improves spontaneously), which may last for months or years. Usually we cannot predict the pattern. During acute attacks, the patient is feverish and extremely sick. Various drugs have been devised to treat rheumatoid arthritis; at the present time, gold salts are particularly helpful, but are, of course, very expensive.

In children, rheumatoid arthritis is known as Still's disease. It usually affects children under the age of ten and involves the entire spinal column, neck, and hips. Typically, the symptoms include a high fever with a rash and involvement of the hands as well. Juvenile rheumatoid arthritis is extremely serious; it usually leads to marked growth retardation and spontaneous bony fusion of the major joints in the hips and lower spine.

Marie-Strümpell Disease

Rheumatoid arthritis in men is a severe condition known as ankylosing spondylitis or Marie Strümpell disease (Fig. 4–3B). It is a progressive, inflammatory arthritis that attacks the back in particular and is seen almost exclusively in young men between the ages of twenty and forty. Typically the rib cage is affected first, and bony growths fuse the ribs to the vertebrae. Fusion stops the normal bellows action of the rib cage itself. Normally, the ribs expand the chest by almost two inches during inhalation; in patients with Marie-Strümpell disease, the rib cage rarely expands more than a half inch.

Reduced rib expansion is the first physical finding that alerts the physician to the almost certain presence of this terrible form of arthritis. X rays will usually reveal marked bony formation directly across the front of the vertebrae, with complete infiltration of bone over the ligaments that support the spine. After a while the spine becomes so stiff that the patient walks with a peculiar forward hunched-over posture; in X rays the spine resembles a bamboo pole to such a degree that it is called bamboo spine. There is no question that there is a genetic predisposition to this disease in men, just as there is a predisposition to rheumatoid arthritis in women. It is also known that blacks in Africa rarely get the disease, while North American Indians contract it as frequently as Caucasian males in this country.

There is no miracle cure for Marie-Strümpell disease. The same basic treatment of heat, rest, and salicylates that is used for rheumatoid arthritis in women is recommended and occasionally will bring some relief. Patients with arthritic disorders who live in a warm, dry climate usually are much happier and have less pain than those who live on the Eastern seaboard in a cold, damp region.

CONGENITAL DISORDERS

Congenital conditions are those with which you are born. Congenital conditions are not necessarily genetic or hereditary, but are caused by some type of malformation or something that went wrong during the time that the new human being was growing inside the womb. Some congenital conditions are extremely mild—for example, a birthmark or an unusual mole. Others can be incredibly disastrous: Infants can be born with two heads, an extra limb, or with the entire spinal cord open with the spinal nerve roots showing. Fortunately, children with some of the more severe conditions do not live; often they are stillborn or die shortly after birth. In fact, the fetuses in approximately seventy percent of all miscarriages are malformed and would have been grossly abnormal had they been born. Naturally, there are too many congenital conditions to describe in detail, and only those that are of significance to your back are listed.

Transitional Vertebrae

One of the most significant congenital conditions in the lower lumbar spine is that of transitional vertebrae. Normally, there are five lumbar vertebrae stacked directly above the sacrum, as mentioned in the section on anatomy. Occasionally, however, there are only four lumbar vertebrae because the fifth has been incorporated in the sacrum. This condition is known as *sacralization of lumbar five*. In other cases, there are six lumbar vertebrae instead of five, and then we talk about *lumbarization of the first sacral vertebra*. If there are either four, five, or six vertebrae in the lumbar spine and there are no abnormalities in the facet joints that unite one vertebra to the other, then there rarely is significant trouble. However, as has been shown in some studies, people with six lumbar vertebrae have a longer trunk and therefore seem to put more stresses on their lumbosacral joint, with more back pain in life.

One of the more significant congenital problems occurs when the transverse process, the little arm that comes out from each side of the lumbar vertebrae (Fig. 1–3), actually touches the sacrum on one side to form a transitional lumbosacral vertebra. Many times a joint forms in that area which creates abnormal motions, or torque, and causes unusual stresses and pressures on the discs and nerve roots, usually at the level above the transitional vertebrae (see Fig. 4–10).

In a recent study which I did with Dr. Robert Durning, we examined twelve patients who had transitional vertebrae; all of them had significant problems at the disc space above the affected vertebra. All twelve needed surgery for decompression of the nerve roots one level above the transitional vertebrae, and they also needed a spinal fusion (welding of the vertebrae together) as well.

Facet Tropism—Asymmetry

The next type of congenital disorder is called facet tropism. This is a relatively common condition in which the little facet joints toward the back of each vertebra are abnormally aligned in the spine. Most of the time, in the lower lumbar spine, the facet joints are lined up so that one is directly in contact with the other, as though they were shaking hands. However, when the facet is twisted so that the joint is aligned *horizontally* instead of *vertically* (facet tropism), abnormal stresses are produced at that joint (Fig. 1–3). This causes abnormal spinal mechanics and, over a period of many years, can lead to increasing back pain. Facet tropism is extremely common, however, and is routinely seen on X rays of people who do not have any type of back pain. If there is no pain, the tropism is of no significance, but occasionally a tropism can cause marked symptoms. I'm sure that these are the conditions that can be so successfully treated with manipulation, especially when the facets tend to slip out of place or sublux.

Spina Bifida

This congenital condition is an incomplete closure of the posterior bony elements of the vertebrae at the lower lumbar spine

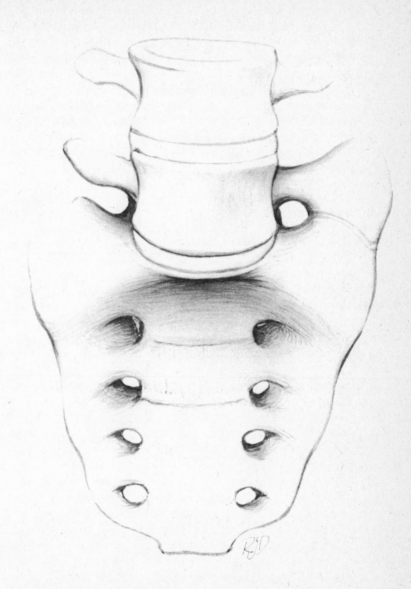

Figure 4–10. This is a drawing of the lower two lumbar vertebrae on top of the sacrum. As seen on the right, the transverse process is touching the sacrum and produces an abnormal joint at that point. This sets up abnormal stresses which are transmitted to disc spaces both above and below that area, and can lead to disc derangement and degeneration. The condition is called a transitional vertebra.

or sacrum. It occurs so frequently that it is almost a variant of "normal." When it cannot be noticed externally and is purely an X-ray finding, it is called spina bifida occulta. It does not weaken the spine; in fact, some of our greatest athletes have this condition.

In rare cases the spinal defect is much greater, and the spinal cord or nerves actually protrude, causing profound nerve deficit and paralysis of the lower extremities. These severe conditions are almost always noted at birth.

Although spina bifida occulta figures prominently in legal cases—especially rear-end auto accidents—it has almost no medical significance.

PSYCHONEUROTIC PROBLEMS

It is now known that many people with low back pain are victims of severe stress. Our society is rife with financial and family-related stresses that can cause people to develop disease symptoms and actual disorders. Stomach ulcers are a perfect example. They are often found in high-strung individuals who are always hurrying to meet increasing demands on their time. The ulcer that develops can be seen on X ray, and certainly is not something that is imagined. However, the patient would probably not have the ulcer if it were not for a terrible marital problem, miserable job, or stressful commute in very congested traffic. Sometimes eliminating the underlying stress with a change in jobs or a solution to the marital discord will make the ulcer disappear.

Previous studies have shown that there are two types of people. The Type A person is high-strung, hyperactive, and ulcer-prone; he tends to have high blood pressure and be extremely anxious and tense. The Type B individual is usually more relaxed and less compulsive; he tends to relax and enjoy life more. The Type B individual enjoys his leisure activities and sports, and rarely gets too worked up or upset about schedules or deadlines. There is no question that Type B people tend to outlive Type A people and that stresses take their toll on the Type A group. If you are a Type A person, it is hard to change your genetic and environmental makeup, but you can try to reduce stress in your daily life. Actually most people have a mixture of Type A and Type B characteristics.

The Hysterical Patient

It has been proven that people can imagine certain problems, whether they be abdominal pain, headaches, or backaches. Imagined pain is some people's way of dealing with stress they do not wish to recognize on a conscious basis. The pain they feel is real, although there is no organic basis for it. *They are not malingering* or consciously mimicking symptoms for financial or other secondary gains. The hysterical patient's back pain can be severe, but it is the product of anxiety and improper psychological defense mechanisms rather than the product of an actual spinal disorder. Anxiety causes muscle spasms, which lead to severe muscle tension and pain. Tension and pain in turn lead to more anxiety and more muscle tension and pain. The vicious cycle thus set up can lead to recurrent back problems of a serious nature.

Most hysterical patients are females who are greatly agitated and unable to deal with the stress under which they have been placed. They usually have severe back pain that radiates "all over the body." Words like *excruciating* are frequently used to describe the severity of the symptoms. These patients usually say they have pain in every single muscle and bone of their body; in some cases, they actually claim that they are totally paralyzed. The patient usually demands to be seen immediately and often is brought to the doctor's office in an ambulance or is carried in by relatives. These gestures are an attempt by the patient to emphasize the severity of the pain and show a deep psychological need for help.

The physician should suspect hysteria when the patient enters his office and flatters him for his reputation, while at the same time degrading all previous physicians who have rendered treatment. Hysterical patients will imply that their previous physicians were incompetent since they were unable to help them or diagnose their problem. Although they flatter the new doctor, the wary doctor realizes that sooner or later he will be added to her list of inept physicians because the *proper diagnosis in these cases is the last thing the patient wants to hear.*

Usually during the history taking, many hidden causes for the patient's anxiety, such as family problems or severe work-related difficulties, are uncovered. Usually the patient's sex life is extremely disturbed, and her husband may be having an affair with another woman. Sometimes the patient herself may have become involved in some type of love triangle and is greatly troubled. Her back pain is a good subconscious way to get out of the problem without directly confronting it. The patient sometimes states that touching her causes severe pain and it is impossible for her to have sexual relations.

Although the hysterical patient complains of severe pain, she usually has a very flat facial expression, called *la belle indifference*, that belies the "excruciating" pain she is experiencing. Patients with hysteria usually have very bizarre reactions to the physical examination. Their neurological reactions do not in any way follow the normal patterns of nerve distribution, and any reasonably trained physician can usually diagnose hysteria immediately (Fig. 4–11A). Reflexes are grossly exaggerated, and numbness in the hands and feet is so bizarre that it is usually present only in the areas that stockings and gloves would cover (stocking-glove anesthesia). This pattern of numbness is neurologically impossible. Vibration from a tuning fork over bony prominences is only felt on one side of the body, another neurologic impossibility.

Hysterical patients also exaggerate the motions of the spine, and therefore it is important for the physician (with a nurse present) to observe the patient while he or she is disrobing to see if motions are exaggerated. Many times while the doctor turns his head, the patient will slip out of stockings or other clothing easily. If the physician asks the patient to bend down to pick up something, however, she will almost always say that it is impossible for her to move at all. These gross contradictions in the patient's disability and the history will usually clinch the diagnosis. Placebos—drugs that have no pharmacologic value— usually give the patient tremendous relief.

The best treatment for the hysterical patient is reassurance and a regimen of mild sedatives or other drugs that cannot cause harm or addiction. It is not wise for the physician to tell the patient that she is hysterical and thereby unmask her situation. These people need their hysteria as a crutch to control the tremendous amount of anxiety they have. If the physician takes away the patient's mask of hysteria, other symptoms—like heart palpitations or headaches—will usually replace the back pain, and the problem will only be compounded. A very kind and understanding physician can be of great help to these patients, and can usually assist them with family, marital, or work-related problems until their stressful episode is solved and

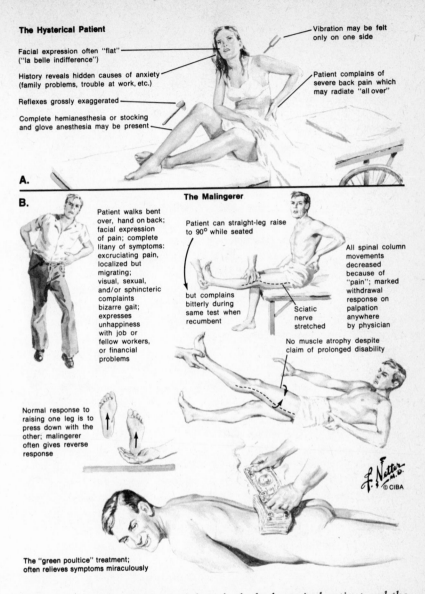

The Hysterical Patient

Vibration may be felt only on one side

Facial expression often "flat" ("la belle indifference")

History reveals hidden causes of anxiety (family problems, trouble at work, etc.)

Reflexes grossly exaggerated

Complete hemianesthesia or stocking and glove anesthesia may be present

Patient complains of severe back pain which may radiate "all over"

A.

B.

The Malingerer

Patient walks bent over, hand on back; facial expression of pain; complete litany of symptoms: excruciating pain, localized but migrating; visual, sexual, and/or sphincteric complaints bizarre gait; expresses unhappiness with job or fellow workers, or financial problems

Patient can straight-leg raise to 90° while seated

but complains bitterly during same test when recumbent

Sciatic nerve stretched

All spinal column movements decreased because of "pain"; marked withdrawal response on palpation anywhere by physician

No muscle atrophy despite claim of prolonged disability

Normal response to raising one leg is to press down with the other; malingerer often gives reverse response

The "green poultice" treatment; often relieves symptoms miraculously

Figure 4–11. This illustration defines both the hysterical patient and the malingerer. The hysterical patient actually has symptoms and pains that are real. However, they occur because of inner stresses and anxieties, which cause these symptoms. The imagined pain is the patient's way of dealing with stress that the patient cannot recognize on a conscious basis. The pain felt is real, but there is no organic or physical basis for it. The malingerer, however, is consciously trying to fake pain and disability because of secondary gain involved. Malingerers usually respond miraculously to the "green poultice" treatment. (Copyright © 1980, CIBA Pharmaceutical Company)

their symptoms spontaneously subside. In more severe cases, psychiatric referral is necessary. It is unwise to admit these patients to a hospital or to prescribe braces or corsets; these actions only reinforce their neuroses and convince the patient that something really is seriously wrong.

The Hypochondriac

Hypochondriasis is the imaginary belief that you have a certain illness or disease. It is very common in both male and female medical students. As they learn about various diseases, some medical students actually start to believe they have them. It is sometimes almost impossible to convince them otherwise. Hypochondriasis is more common in women, especially in neglected housewives who are bored while their husbands are away at work. They have little to occupy their time and start to imagine various illnesses until they are convinced they have some disease. As more and more women enter the work force and people have less time on their hands, hypochondriasis is likely to be more equally distributed between the sexes.

Hypochondriacs spend a great deal of their lives trading in one set of symptoms for another. One month they have headache problems and see various doctors to have the headaches diagnosed and treated. The next month they will consult someone for gynecologic problems and menstrual irregularity. Several months later they will have back pain, which they find difficult to control. They will almost challenge the physician to make the proper diagnosis. These patients have a tremendous need to be sick and usually also have severe neuroses, which may be either temporary or permanent, depending on their cause. Some people with hypochondriasis undergo three or four operations on their back. They are actually masochistic; they have a psychological need to experience pain.

Hypochondriacs go from doctor to doctor looking for a cure, and usually after two or three operations they are, unfortunately, hooked on medications, especially tranquilizing and pain-relieving drugs. The unwary physician can fall victim to these patients and add more prescriptions to the pile. I have met patients who take eight or ten different types of medication daily—one patient told me that she took over sixty pills a day to relieve her pain and anxiety! Tranquilizers are prescribed much too readily for people with low back pain. Addiction to Librium, Valium, and other tranquilizing agents is an extremely serious problem in this country, and is a result of prescribing abuse by physicians. It is all to easy to get rid of an anxious and tense hypochondriac with a prescription. A physician giving good medical care will withhold the prescription and attempt to recognize why the patient is a hypochondriac instead. The problem can sometimes be solved by a mutual understanding between the rest of the family and the physician, and by proper education of the patient. However, in some situations psychiatric counseling is required for a permanent cure.

The cost of hypochondriasis to our society is extremely high. Many millions of dollars each year are lost by employers and companies who have to pay for the numerous doctor and hospital visits these patients arrange. In addition to undergoing repeated "unsuccessful" operations for relief of their pain, some of these patients quit work, live on unemployment compensation insurance, and become dependent at home. Hypochondriacs often have unhappy marriages and problems with their children. Usually their lives are so painful that they imagine medical symptoms in order to cope. They journey from therapist to chiropractor, and from physician to physician, in search of some form of help.

Fortunately, pain clinics are springing up throughout the country where the *entire* patient's problems are treated. These clinics practice holistic medicine, meaning they treat the patient as a whole, rather than a related series of signs and symptoms. Unfortunately, in our society, medicine is geared toward the patient who already has a sickness or illness; we try to cure symptoms *after* they are present and fully developed. In Far Eastern cultures, the aim of medicine is to *prevent* illness. The emphasis in this country is rapidly shifting toward the Far Eastern concept of preventive medicine and toward holistic care. Large family-practice groups are forming throughout the United States to take care of all the patient's needs rather than specific, isolated illnesses.

It is most important to break the hypochondriac's drug habit before addiction occurs. Pain clinics have developed very clever ways to wean the patients from their medications. Tranquilizer and sedative use is gradually reduced and then stopped. (Narcotic addicts are switched to methadone or clonidine, which are less addictive and safer. The dosage is then tapered so that the patient is completely weaned from all drugs.) When the patient's drug dose is reduced to practically nothing, many clinics substitute a placebo for several days. The patient then realizes that he can control his pain without medication for it. The technique usually works well if the patient is given proper counseling and emotional support.

The hypochondriac is extremely difficult to treat—he usually becomes frustrated with his physician, and his physician often becomes upset and exasperated with him. It is helpful to spell out certain ground rules in the beginning so that both the physician and patient can agree on goals and expectations. Patients have a right to be informed about their condition and should be given as bright a prognosis as possible. The physician must be open and helpful, and should be readily available during times of emergency or serious emotional stress. The doctor has the right to expect the patient to follow through with physical therapy, vocational rehabilitation, weight control regimens, and exercise programs, and to practice self-control when it comes to medication.

The patient also has a right to tell the physician about serious psychological and personal problems without having the physician reject these issues as unimportant or irrelevant. If the physician feels that psychological or psychiatric help is needed, the patient should be able to accept this advice without becoming insulted.

Pain clinics use many proven techniques, including neurosurgery, electrical stimulation, biofeedback, hypnosis, nerve blocks, muscle relaxation training, spinal injections, dietary instructions, psychotherapy, psychiatric care, acupuncture, physical therapy, and withdrawal of medications. Some treatments must be done in the hospital, but most can be performed on an outpatient basis. Clinics are located in most major cities throughout the United States, and the well-informed physician will be able to refer his patients to a local treatment center (see Chapter 9).

In pain clinics the goals set for each patient include a *treatment goal* and an *occupational goal*, as well as an attempt to establish better family and personal relationships. Each patient formulates his own goals and is told exactly what to expect from hospitalization and treatment. Most patients treated in pain-control clinics are extremely pleased with their care. Very few patients finish a treatment program without having made some advancement in the control of their pain.

I have made several references to patients being placed on placebos. Patients are given certain innocuous drugs, which they think are effective medications. Granted, this practice is deceptive, but frankly, it helps most patients and rids many of serious drug addiction problems.

All medications exhibit what is called the placebo effect. Almost any form of treatment for back pain will generally cure approximately one third of patients. The fact that a third of all medications given will relieve pain whether or not they have been proven effective in clinical trials shows that the psychological benefits of a medicine are extremely potent. The psychological benefit acts in a way similar to the laying on of the hands used by kings in earlier times. A similar effect is obtained by faith healers. This psychological benefit is, in essence, what the placebo effect is all about. Since one third of people have pain with psychological overtones, many can experience great relief by merely having profound belief in the power of either a medication or a certain doctor. People who think they are going to die when they go in the hospital often do! Others survive extremely severe, life-threatening illnesses against all odds because they have extremely strong psychological control and have been able to affect their physical status by sheer will power.

A natural substance found in the human body, especially in the pituitary gland, explains some of the placebo effect. *Beta-endorphin*, a morphine like substance produced by the nerve cells, acts as the body's own internal painkiller. In some medical centers in this country, neurosurgeons have placed electrodes in the brain and the spine; these electrodes have then been used to transmit radio signals to the patient's brain to release beta-endorphin in minute quantities. Soon after this stimulation, some people experience relief from chronic back pain, which lasts from a few hours to several days. As science advances, and knowledge about drugs such as beta-endorphin grows, we will probably learn how to extract chemicals that can be used to treat pain from our nervous system or from the nervous system of animals.

One form of beta-endorphin is called enkephalin. We know that some people tend to secrete more enkephalin than others. Investigations are presently under way to determine exactly what areas of the body these chemicals stimulate, and how we can control their secretion.

I have always been amazed by the range of pain tolerance in my patients. Some require almost no pain medication after surgery, while others need extremely large doses of painkilling drugs. When I was training at The Shriner's Hospital in Winnipeg, Canada, in 1962 and 1963, we treated a great number of Canadian Indians. These patients were so stoic that they rarely had pain of any kind. Even after major operations they often went without even a single injection of any painkilling drug. Some patients had spine fusions one day and the next day got out of bed and walked almost without any pain. Conversely, I've had patients from other ethnic groups who are extremely emotional and labile. They exhibit hyperactive responses to normal situations that would not excite other people. Very emotional, excitable people tend to experience greater pain than do stoics like the Canadian and American Indians, and thus usually require large amounts of painkillers and sedatives.

Compensatory Low Back Pain—The Malingerer

The malingerer is a person, generally a male, who complains of low back pain, but has a conscious secondary gain in mind, a gain that can be absolutely real or merely imagined. These patients actually are aware that they are trying to defraud someone, but may try to justify their actions. They feel that their employer "owes it" to them, or that they have been maligned in some other way by the company they work for, the government, or some other organ of society. They are not like the hysterical patient who has totally unconscious motivation and does not understand the reason for his or her symptoms at all.

It is important to remember that a patient who is malingering can be completely disinterested in financial rewards. He may be seeking other compensation, either in the form of an easier job or some type of retribution for ills done to himself or his family. In contrast, the compensatory patient who is malingering is interested in monetary gain. He is looking for some type of settlement, either as a result of an injury at work or because of some grievance. Malingerers can have compensatory low back pain, but the two terms are not always synonymous.

The patient with compensatory pain in his back usually has a typical history. Often he has already seen a lawyer before visiting his physician, and he is usually reluctant to divulge the amount for which he is suing. In fact, many times the patients will tell you "frankly" that they are not at all interested in financial gain, but only want to find the cause of their pain and be rid of it. Of course, this is totally untrue; the patient has already been well instructed by his lawyer not to discuss the amount of the suit with the physician or anyone else.

Sometimes the patient has been in an accident, either while at work or in a motor vehicle. He may be trying to collect compensation from his employer or from an insurance company over a prolonged period. If a patient claims injury on the job, a careful questioning will usually reveal anger with a fellow worker or with a supervisor. Sometimes the patient has been threatened with a layoff and finds that feigning a back injury will help him keep the job or at least earn him compensation for the real or imagined injustices he has suffered.

Many patients who have been involved in rear-end automobile accidents and have a suit pending complain of severe neck pain (referred to as a whiplash injury). Whiplash can occur if a person is sitting relaxed in a car parked at a stoplight and is struck from behind. The victim's head whips back and forth on his relatively fragile neck, and he suffers severe muscle sprains, with protracted neck aches and pain. Severe whiplash will cause injuries that can be seen on neck X rays, and the patient will show specific diagnostic indications of the injury. Unfortunately, in addition to the many ethical practicing lawyers, there are some greedy and unethical people in the legal profession. They have distorted their clients' minds with tales of enormous financial settlements after some minor accident. As a result, patients will sometimes claim ridiculous disabilities as an outcome of their injury. Those who seek this form of compensation suffer from what I call the green poultice syndrome. I use this term to refer to patients who respond miraculously to the figurative application of hundred-dollar bills over the area of their back that hurts most. When the green poultice is thick enough, their pain mysteriously disappears and they are cured! (See Fig. 4–11B.)

Occasionally, unscrupulous lawyers who make their living on contingency fees or on percentages of their client's settlement become ambulance chasers. They will try to talk accident victims into suing *anyone* who could even remotely be considered a guilty party. In most states, legal fees are limited to a certain low percentage of the settlement, but in others they may go as high as 50 percent. Some lawyers coach their clients, teaching them an entire litany of signs and symptoms. I have even seen twelve- and fourteen-year-old children who have memorized medical and legal terms that could not possibly have been in their vocabulary prior to their accident (or to their visit to the lawyer).

Many compensatory patients will recount a history of severe disability that includes blurred vision, ringing in the ears, or a decrease in bowel function or sexual activity since the accident. However, despite coaching, the patient usually has bizarre findings that are not at all consistent with the claimed symptoms. Usually he walks with an increased lumbar lordosis and decreased range of motion in the entire spine. After bending forward, the patient usually returns to the erect position with such stiff motion that he is said to have "cogwheel rigidity." This is usually a definitive sign to an astute physician.

Malingerers are trying to confuse the examiner, to cloud his opinion of what is wrong. They are consciously trying to make their situation worse than it actually is. Because most patients are not really good actors, it is usually easy to diagnose the malingerer correctly. His complaints rarely coincide with the symptoms he describes.

What does the physician do when he suspects malingering? The worst thing would be to confront the patient directly and tell him that he is faking. It is almost impossible to prove malingering beyond the shadow of a doubt since pain is such a personal and subjective experience. The best course for the physician is to state that *no organic basis can be found for the patient's symptoms.* Most insurance companies, employers, and ethical lawyers immediately understand the significance of this statement, and will do everything they can to discourage the patient from pursuing further legal or compensatory action.

In general, patients with psychoneurotic problems are a sorry group and require a great amount of care and attention. The physician must try to be compassionate and understand that they are often desperate, either because of emotional disability or because of severe financial burdens. It is wrong for the physician to play God and judge the patient harshly. The physician can be more helpful if he tries to be understanding and help the patient come to a socially acceptable solution to his problem.

TOXICITY

The term *toxicity* is used to refer to some form of poisoning. We live in a society where many things we once took for granted, such as our air and water, can actually be harmful for our bodies. As mentioned later in the discussion of malignant tumors, industrial pollutants—which we have been breathing for many years—can cause serious poisoning, lead to heavy metal intoxication, and in some cases cause various forms of cancer. Industrial wastes can also pollute rivers and contaminate the fish that inhabit those rivers. Fortunately, our government is now taking steps to stop pollution.

Examples of heavy metal poisoning are the cases of women who were given radium for conditions such as high blood pressure and arthritis in the 1930s and 1940s. At that time, radium treatment was considered to be an important form of health care. These patients later developed radium intoxication of the bones that resulted in tumors and other life-threatening conditions. During this same era, many workers who applied luminous paint to watch dials were exposed to heavy metals. They repeatedly ingested minute quantities of radium as a result of touching the tip of their paintbrush to their tongue to make a fine point on the brush. Twenty to thirty years later, they were found to have radium poisoning! Unfortunately, toxic conditions can take many years to surface, and by that time the result of the industrial blunders usually cannot be reversed.

The use of lead in paint has been a problem of great concern, especially since small children ingest lead that chips off the walls and furniture in their homes. This type of lead intoxication is particularly common in low-income-housing projects, where lead-based paint has been used for years. Fortunately, pediatricians are now very aware of this condition and lead paint is no longer available.

TUMORS

Tumors are abnormal growths in the body. We do not understand why tumors grow; fortunately, most tumors around the
spine are benign, or not cancerous.

Benign Tumors: Not Cancerous

Benign tumors can occur in the nerve roots themselves or in the
coverings of the spinal cord (the meninges). These tumors
usually are not serious and are quite rare. When they occur, they
can cause pressure or pain. A very astute physician may be able
to diagnose these conditions by physical examination and
history alone, but usually it requires very elaborate laboratory
and other diagnostic tests which we will describe later.

Other benign tumors in the spine occur in the bones
themselves and can be part of the vertebrae. A good example
would be a small tumor called an osteoid osteoma. It is benign
and characteristically causes severe pain, especially at night.
The pain usually wakens the patient because of its piercing
character, and the patient almost always obtains relief directly
by taking aspirin. The diagnosis is not too difficult to make, as
special X rays and radioactive bone scans usually "light up" the
tumor. Total surgical removal almost always results in a complete cure.

Another common benign tumor causing back pain is the
lipoma. Lipomas are small, fatty tumors found outside of the
fascia surrounding the muscles. They slip back and forth between the skin and muscle bundles of the spine and can be felt
by the examiner. Lipomas can cause severe localized back pain,
but this can often be alleviated with injections of local anesthesia and cortisone-type drugs. Lipomas that continue to increase
in size may have to be surgically removed.

Fortunately, benign tumors rarely become life-threatening, but they can cause severe nerve root pressure, especially
when they grow inside the spinal canal where the nerve roots
run. If the tumors are up in the thoracic or cervical spinal
region, they can be more serious, even though benign, because
as they increase in size, they exert pressure directly on the spinal
cord and can thus lead to muscle weakness and even paralysis.
Orthopaedists know that severe pain when the patient lies down

usually indicates the presence of a tumor. Almost all other kinds of back pain are markedly relieved when the patient lies down and reduces the stresses of gravity.

Malignant Tumors: Cancerous

The counterpart of the benign, less serious, tumor is the malignant tumor. These tumors are always serious. They can begin in the spine as an intrinsic part of the bones or nerves themselves (a primary tumor), or they can spread (metastasize) to the spine from another location (a secondary tumor). The most common primary bone tumor in the entire body is a *multiple myeloma*, a very malignant tumor that is most common inside the spine, especially in the bodies of the vertebrae. It is most often seen in the thoracic or the lumbar spine and usually occurs in people over the age of fifty. Fortunately there are now many drugs and other medications that are effective in relieving the pain from multiple myeloma, and which may also, in some instances, effect a cure or prolonged remission (a period of relative freedom from tumor symptoms). In addition to primary bone tumors there are also primary nerve-root tumors that can occur either in the nerves themselves or in the coverings of the spinal cord (the meninges). Fortunately, these tumors are quite rare.

Unfortunately, malignant tumors in humans are becoming increasingly more common. We now know, as was mentioned before, that heredity plays an incredibly important role in malignant tumors. If a woman's ancestors had breast cancer, her chances of having breast cancer are extremely high. This is also true of certain other types of cancers, and a hereditary predisposition to having a certain type of tumor—along with certain abuses to which we subject our bodies—will stack the cards against us. We know that people living in certain states in America have a much higher cancer rate than those who live in other states. Higher rates usually occur in industrial areas where air pollution is high. Pollution of the air with asbestos fibers and other types of residues from industrial smoke also appears to cause lung cancer. It has also been known for years, and there is absolutely no question on this point, that cigarette smoking in large amounts will eventually lead to lung cancer. At the Columbia-Presbyterian Medical Center, where I have the privilege of working, there are approximately five hundred physicians; of those who used to smoke almost 95 percent have now stopped because they have seen with their own eyes that *cigarette smoking definitely does increase the risk of lung cancer!*

So in effect, then, we not only have a hereditary predisposition toward malignant tumors, but we also can acquire certain malignant tumors through our environment and by abusing our bodies. The most common tumors that spread to the skeleton (especially to the spine) come from the breast, prostate gland, kidneys, lungs, and the thyroid gland in the neck. Characteristically, these tumors have special modes of behavior; for example, tumors that spread to the spine (metastasize) usually replace bone and form what we call lytic tumors. These tumors usually replace bony material in the vertebrae. After a while the spine will tend to fracture and collapse, causing secondary compression fractures. The fractures are a direct result of weakening by the tumor and are not related to any other abnormality in the spine.

Tumors of the kidney, lung, and thyroid many times act very much like breast tumors; they tend to replace bone and show as areas of bony destruction on X rays of the spine.

Tumors of the prostate gland—which are, of course, only in males—also tend to spread to the spine, but instead of eating away bone, they deposit more bone in the spine. Characteristically, these tumors cause vertebrae to look dense on an X ray. Tumors that lay down new bone are called osteoblastic.

Secondary tumors can usually be diagnosed by certain laboratory tests and other types of X-ray techniques, such as computerized scanning of the skeleton. It is the primary, or original, cancer in the body that must be found and cured, if at all possible, in order to slow the activity and growth of the secondary tumors (the metastases).

Unfortunately, at this time most major malignant tumors are ultimately fatal unless diagnosed early, when they can often be completely cured. With modern diagnostic and therapeutic techniques, people are able to live much longer and with a greatly improved quality of life than ever before.

Five
SELF-DIAGNOSIS AND SELF-HELP FOR YOUR PAINFUL BACK

EARLY SIGNS: HEED THE WARNING

Most back pain comes on rather slowly. Usually there will be some early warning signs, generally in the form of muscle twitches or aches that are present several days before disabling pain occurs. However, when a person who is out of shape engages in too-strenuous activity, such as moving furniture or playing many sets of tennis, the pain will usually occur that afternoon or the next morning, and can be most acute. Instantaneous, severe pain can also follow the most ordinary nonstrenuous actions, such as bending over to put on trousers. In these cases, the motion somehow triggers severe muscle spasms along the spine.

Pain that precedes a back problem is usually localized to one area—for example, the lower spine on either the right or left side or the region of the sacroiliac joint. Pain may also follow the course of a nerve, traveling around the chest wall and underneath the ribs, directly to the shoulders, or down the upper or lower extremities. Some patients experience pain only at night. Although night pain can be a significant diagnostic sign, it is usually caused by a poor mattress or poor sleeping posture.

In addition to pain, there are usually other signals of an impending back problem. Sometimes certain muscle groups and even the fingers and toes will be weak. (Weakness can be an indication of a very serious condition, and a physician should be consulted immediately.) Numbness and tingling are other rather frequent signals. They usually indicate that nerves are being compressed or pinched and that something is interfering with the normal conduction of nerve impulses. Often, people with arthritic changes in their back and spondylosis (degenerative changes, see page 48) will be stiff when they wake up. After they get going, they loosen up and can pursue normal activities. (A warm tub bath first thing in the morning will usually relieve this type of stiffness.)

Other signs that can signal a serious problem are unexplained weight loss and blood in the stools. Bright red blood can either be the result of bleeding hemorrhoids or of a tumor inside the rectum. Blood from a condition high inside the digestive tract, such as a bleeding ulcer, usually is black in color and produces stools that look like tar and lead to diarrhea. Both of these signs may indicate serious conditions, and a physician should be promptly consulted, especially if you are also experiencing loss of appetite, muscle wasting, and weakness.

WHAT TO DO ON YOUR OWN

Whether the early warning signals are mild muscular twinges or severe disabling pain, you must heed them and take immediate action. Most patients who have low back pain, whether it is of the slowly progressing variety or the severely intense type, can help themselves greatly by first of all going to bed. Generally, "Take it easy" is the best advice to give a patient. Ninety-five percent of all aches and pains in the back will respond to bed rest and *warm* tub baths. Baths should be taken at least twice a day for approximately twenty minutes. The water should be *warm, not hot,* since some people have poor temperature-regulating mechanisms and can burn themselves easily. Heat of any kind is useful, but should be applied with care. Moist heat may feel better to an individual, but has not been proven to be more effective than dry heat. If a heating pad is used in bed, be careful not to fall asleep on it since severe burns can occur, especially if the pad is not wrapped in a towel. If you want to nap while using a heating pad, have someone wake you after twenty or thirty minutes. Other heating devices, such as a hydrocollator (a pad filled with a heat-retaining material) or even an old-fashioned hot water bottle, are also most helpful. These devices are heated prior to application. Again, caution is necessary to prevent burns, especially if you have insensitive skin. After two or three days, some people find that alternating cold (ice packs) and heat over the area of muscle spasm provides greater relief than heat alone.

Bed rest should be taken on a firm mattress with a pillow positioned underneath the head and back. The most comfortable posture is a semisitting position; it is obtained by putting another pillow under the legs at the knee. You can also take "bed" rest on a couch, again in the semisitting position. Keeping the hips and knees bent, with a small support underneath the head and in the small of the back takes most of the pressure off the spine and helps resolve muscle spasm.

A little bit of brandy or another form of alcohol may be taken as a mild sedative if desired. Alcohol in moderate amounts can be soothing and ease muscle spasm and tension. As has been discussed, emotional stress has a great deal to do with backaches. Having a drink or two can be more than just mildly helpful, especially if back pain has been triggered by an emotional crisis.

After about eight to ten days of bed rest and heat applications, you should be improving. This is the time to start a gentle exercise program. Begin with the six PREs (Pain-Relieving Exercises) described in Chapter 3. Unlike the five KPEs (Keim Preventive Exercises), which are designed to prevent back pain, these six exercises are to be done once you have back pain. Begin exercising a week or two after the injury—*never* while the pain is still acute. This will give the muscles and ligaments time to heal. Start the program at a very slow pace, increasing the repetitions by one every second or third day.

It is also important to avoid the type of activity that caused your back pain to begin with. As obvious as this seems, it's worth mentioning. It's amazing how many people will attempt to do chores themselves even though they have suffered back pain recently as a result of similar activities.

Anyone who has read the early portions of this book is aware that the three main causes of back pain are stress,

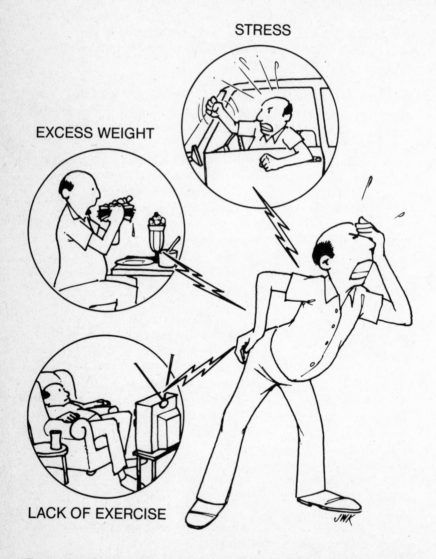

Figure 5–1. The three main contributors to low back pain. They are stress, excess weight, and lack of exercise. (© Columbia University, 1981)

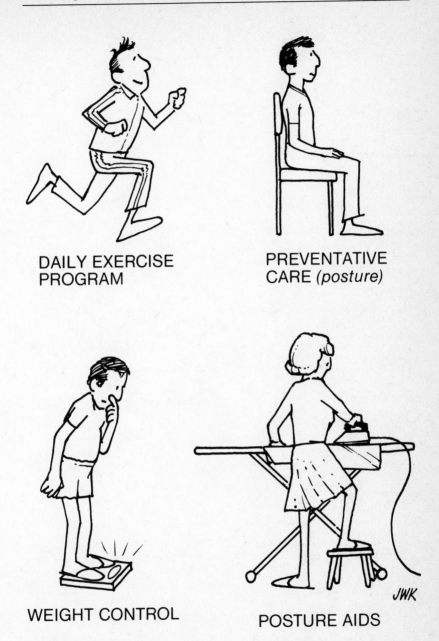

DAILY EXERCISE
PROGRAM

PREVENTATIVE
CARE *(posture)*

WEIGHT CONTROL

POSTURE AIDS

JWK

Figure 5–2. To help prevent back pain, it is best to start a daily exercise program. Watch your weight, use posture aids, and prevent problems by using correct posture. (© Columbia University 1981)

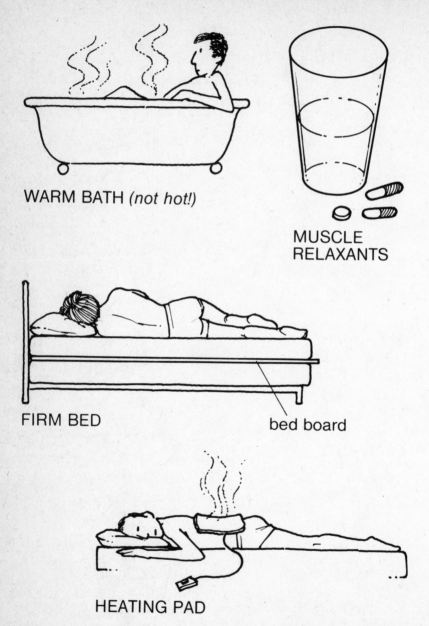

WARM BATH *(not hot!)*

MUSCLE
RELAXANTS

FIRM BED   bed board

HEATING PAD

*Figure 5–3. Some of the aids that can help you when you have back pain.
Use a warm tub (not hot), a firm mattress with a bed board, a heating pad,
and muscle relaxants if prescribed by your doctor. (© Columbia University
1981)*

improper diet, and poor muscle tone or hypokinesis (Fig. 5–1). Therefore, it is important to begin a proper exercise program (the PREs) as soon as possible and to start a reducing diet immediately if you are overweight. Learning proper posture is also most important. Try to stand straight, with your tummy flat and your rump tucked underneath you. This posture will decrease lumbar lordosis and swayback and ensure that the pelvis rests directly below the spine (Fig. 5–2).

Seat supports in your car may be helpful. These can be obtained from most auto supply stores. In fact, special orthopaedic seats are now available from almost all auto dealers. These seats and supports are extremely helpful to people with back problems. The new swivel seat that can be installed in the driver and passenger sides of the front are also useful. They twist so you can get in and out of the car without having to contort your body to slide under the steering wheel or into the passenger's seat. A steering wheel that tilts can also make it easier to get in and out of the car, especially if you are a big person.

Be sure to insert a bed board between the mattress and the box spring of your bed. You may also want to experiment with gel or water beds. Some people find these more satisfactory than an extra-firm mattress. Gel beds, especially those that have a heating element built in (marvelous on cold winter nights), can be most helpful, specifically for people with arthritic spines.

Attention to sitting habits and use of proper chairs at home and especially at work can be most important for the prevention of future backaches. Be certain that you have a little footstool or bar to rest your feet on, whether you are ironing, standing at a work counter, or sitting at your desk. Constantly try to change your position after prolonged periods of immobility by shifting your weight from side to side. Avoid situations where you are standing in one position for a long period of time. Most of these suggestions have already been mentioned, but are so important that they merit repetition (Fig. 5–3). If self-diagnosis and self-help does not solve the problem after three or four weeks, it is time to see your doctor.

Six

WHEN TO SEE YOUR DOCTOR AND HOW TO CHOOSE ONE

If you have tried self-diagnosis and self-help and are still in severe pain after two or three weeks, it is time to seek professional help. As mentioned before, you should seek help *immediately* if you have extremely sharp pain radiating down the leg into the foot, or if there is muscle weakness and wasting. So-called "drop foot" is usually caused by direct compression of the nerves of the lumbosacral area and on rare occasions, immediate surgical decompression is necessary.

DIFFERENT TYPES OF PRACTITIONERS—WHOM TO SEE?

The Family Physician

Naturally, the first person to talk to is your own family physician, whether he is a general practitioner or a medical specialist (in most cases an internist, or one who specializes in internal medicine). Often, he already knows your family history and has examined you and other members of your family in the past. He is familiar with your background and previous illnesses. Usually he can do an excellent job of treating more-routine types of back ailments. If he cannot help you, he can almost always suggest the right person for you to contact for further treatment.

The Chiropractor

Chiropractors have trained in special schools teaching chiropractic techniques, but do not have a degree in medicine. They use manipulative techniques but cannot prescribe medications or perform surgery. Nor can they use any type of technique or treatment that invades the body directly. Chiropractors believe strongly that malalignment of the spine, with slipping or maladjustment of the vertebrae, is the cause of a tremendous variety of symptoms. They believe that these symptoms can be cured or improved by adjustments or manipulations that restore the bony structures to their proper alignment. Chiropractors can belong to either the International Chiropractors Association or to the American Chiropractic Association or both. They largely confine themselves to the use of X rays and manual adjustments to correct spinal malalignment. They also use heat, ultrasound, hydrotherapy (treatment techniques using water), occasionally acupuncture, or other devices or methods to aid in diagnosis and treatment.

Chiropractors can often treat the most routine forms of back pain successfully. It is perfectly safe to consult a chiropractor as long as you are careful to select a practitioner who recognizes his limitations and does not attempt diagnostic or therapeutic techniques that require the advanced training of a physician. Rarely, there are chiropractors who will continue spinal manipulations even if the treatment is not working. Sometimes diagnosis and treatment of a spinal cord tumor or other serious medical problem is thus delayed unnecessarily. I have seen patients in whom diagnosis was delayed until the condition was so far advanced that it was too late to save the patient's life. Despite this possibility, I feel that a chiropractor, if carefully chosen, can be of great help in some cases of back pain.

The Acupuncturist

Acupuncture is based on a system of Oriental medicine which holds that health is obtained through the flow of a substance called Chi. Chi is believed to be a form of electromagnetic energy that sends thousands of currents throughout the body. Hundreds of acupuncture points mapped out over the entire body are the centers of Chi energy.

In acupuncture treatment, small needles are inserted at specific acupuncture points which have been mapped out over the centuries by Eastern specialists who are experts in this type of work. Sometimes several needles will be used together at one point. In some instances, the needles are twirled slightly after insertion. Often, a small electric current is also added to the needles; it can cause a dramatic response. The technique is usually completely painless.

Acupuncture points along the back, especially those along the sides of the vertebrae, are called U points. Acupuncturists seem to be able to make direct connection with the nerve centers of the spine through proper placement of needles at the U points and are thus able to relieve pain for many patients with chronic back problems. Often, repeated treatments are needed before pain is relieved.

I have seen dramatic proof of the relief provided by acupuncture in some of my patients. There is no question that some of acupuncture's therapeutic value, like that of many other forms of medicine, is derived from the placebo effect, and from an individual patient's own strong desire to get better. However, no matter how strong that desire is, acupuncture will not be of help if back pain is caused by a severe organic problem, such as a tumor or other systemic disease.

Steven Palos's book, *The Chinese Art of Healing*, is an excellent source of information on this technique. It covers the practice of acupuncture and its philosophy, a derivative of Taoism.

The Osteopathic Physician

Osteopaths are fully trained physicians who have been trained at a school of osteopathic medicine. These schools award a degree of Doctor of Osteopathy (D.O.), rather than the M.D. degree. Many states now allow a doctor of osteopathy to change his D.O. degree to an M.D., because of the common misconception that all osteopathic training is inferior to that received in a standard medical school. This is not necessarily true; there are many excellent osteopaths now practicing. I personally am most impressed with the treatment that osteopaths provide.

Doctors of osteopathy can either work as general practitioners or as specialists. Depending on their degree of expertise, they can train specifically in the musculoskeletal system. Osteopaths most often use manipulative therapy as a means of treatment; however, they can also prescribe drugs and muscle relaxants or use traction, heat, ultrasound, and occasionally perform surgery. At the present time doctors of osteopathy comprise approximately 5 percent of America's physicians, and handle approximately 12 percent of all patient visits.

The Neurologist

A neurologist is a doctor of medicine who has specialized in diseases related to the nervous system. Neurologists must complete extensive training and are usually board certified in their particular field of expertise. To be board certified a physician must pass a rigorous written and oral examination.

A neurologist will usually do a very thorough examination in his office. Depending on the diagnosis, he may then recommend certain diagnostic tests to confirm his opinion before recommending treatment. A neurologist may treat the patient himself or work in conjunction with a physical therapist, physiatrist, neurosurgeon, or orthopaedic surgeon.

The Neurosurgeon

A neurosurgeon is also a doctor of medicine. He too must complete a long period of specialty training in addition to his years of medical school. Usually, a neurosurgeon must spend five years in residency training after medical school, and if he subspecializes in his field, he must train an additional one or two years beyond the five-year residency. Neurosurgeons usually work very closely with neurologists. Often the neurologist will diagnose the specific problem, and if surgical treatment is required, he will then refer the patient to the neurosurgeon. Neurosurgeons specialize in the treatment of disorders of the brain, spinal cord, and peripheral nerves.

The Orthopaedic Surgeon

An orthopaedic surgeon is a doctor of medicine who has completed one year of training in general surgery after medical school and three or four years in orthopaedic training after that. In addition, if he has subspecialized, as I have, he has taken another one or two years of additional training for a total of five to six years of training beyond the four years of medical school.

An orthopaedist specializes in disorders of the musculoskeletal system and its environs. In orthopaedics, as in other fields of medicine, a person can decide to superspecialize in a very narrow area. For example, I treat only spinal problems; even then, I rarely take patients with problems of the cervical spine (neck), but limit my practice mostly to patients with thoracic and lumbar spine disorders. Although I have a large practice, the field of spinal medicine is very limited, representing only a small percentage of the whole of orthopaedic practice. There are about forty-five or fifty orthopaedists in the United States who limit themselves *only* to disorders of the spine. Although we call ourselves orthopaedic surgeons, we really spend a great deal of our time treating patients without surgery. Approximately eight of every ten patients seen in the office do not require surgery of any kind, and can be treated nonoperatively. Orthopaedic surgeons often work closely with neurologists, neurosurgeons, physiatrists, and physical therapists, and will use braces and corsets, other nonoperative techniques, and, if it is indicated, surgery to relieve specific spinal problems.

The Physiatrist

A physiatrist is a doctor of medicine who specializes in *physical medicine*. The physiatrist uses physical means for treating disorders of the musculoskeletal system; he does not perform any type of surgery and usually works in association with a group of physical therapists, who assist in treating his patients. He prescribes exercises, diathermy, heat or ice treatments, ultrasound, and different methods of injection therapy, along with ethyl chloride sprays and exercises to solve musculoskeletal problems. A good physiatrist can be of tremendous help in relieving pain in and around the spine because he treats spinal disorders frequently and is very familiar with them.

The Physical Therapist

A physical therapist has attended a school of physical therapy, usually affiliated with a medical center, and is registered as a certified physical therapist at graduation. He or she is not a doctor of medicine, osteopathy, or a chiropractor. Although physical therapists do not have a medical degree, they are specially trained in exercise, massage, heat treatments, and other techniques used in treating musculoskeletal aches and pains. The physical therapist can be extremely helpful, especially if he works under the direction of a physiatrist or the orthopaedic surgeon who originally made the diagnosis.

HOW TO CHOOSE YOUR DOCTOR

Many people are gravely concerned about how to choose a good doctor. There is genuine reason for concern because today there are numerous "gurus" and quacks who claim to be able to cure any number of illnesses. Quacks also are willing to relieve people of their hard-earned money, if not their pains, and have been around at least since the early Roman era. Unfortunately, the dishonest and unethical are more numerous in every profession today. However, the great majority of men and women practicing medicine have the highest ethical standards. Remember too that what is really important is the physician's skill as a healer, not the number of degrees hanging on his wall.

A doctor's reputation is a good indicator of his skill. A reputation has to build up over a period of ten or twenty years. A good reputation is not something easily earned. Since most ethical physicians do not use any form of advertising (although it is legal to do so at this time), a good reputation is usually spread best by word of mouth.

The first person to ask for a referral to a specialist would be your family doctor. If he cannot help you, then talk to friends and relatives who are satisfied with their doctors. Consulting advertisements, which are now becoming more common, is usually a risky way to find a doctor. Anyone who can afford to pay the advertising fee can run an ad. The ad tells you nothing about the doctor's skills. Not only could the doctor be unethical, but he could also be totally incompetent. Most people wouldn't buy a car from a salesman just because of his advertising gimmicks. Similarly, you shouldn't choose a physician to whom you will entrust your well-being on the basis of a newspaper or television ad. Finally, it is important not to skimp on health care—you only get one body and you must make it last for many years.

The local county medical society or the American Medical Association is usually an excellent reference source for information regarding a specific type of physician. They will usually be happy to give you the names of three or four doctors in your area who can help you with your health problem. Because of the nature of such referral services, they will not tell you if one person is better than another.

You can also consult the *Directory of Medical Specialists*, a publication issued every year that is probably available in your local library. If major surgery is contemplated, you should look through this directory and research your physician or surgeon. There is nothing wrong with investigating the person to whom you are entrusting your health care. The man or woman who will be taking care of your body must not only be above reproach ethically, but also as technically competent as possible. Usually a physician who is associated with a large medical school, and is a professor or on the faculty of that medical school, will be ethical and competent. The finer medical schools will not tolerate incompetents. Especially when choosing a surgeon, check to see if he is board certified in his specialty. Certification indicates that a physician has completed several years of specialty training after medical school, and then—after at least two years of practice—has passed board examinations in his specialty. Board examinations are extremely difficult to pass, and most physicians study four or five years preparing for their Boards.

It is also important to see that your physician has kept up with his medical specialty after he has become board certified. Usually physicians who are writing scientific papers and have published books in their field are the ones who are attuned to the latest developments in their specialty. Try to find out if your physician attends regular meetings of the county and national medical societies, and especially if he has been an officer or has actively participated in those societies. There is also nothing wrong with checking on your doctor's reputation by asking other doctors and nurses you know.

When choosing a surgeon, find out how frequently the physician has performed the specific operation you require and what the results were. Don't be squeamish—ask the doctor directly how often he has done that procedure, and what his good and bad results were. An ethical physician will be perfectly honest with you. When I discuss surgery with patients, I like to put all of the cards on the table and tell them exactly what the chances of success and the risks are. Nothing is to be gained by trying to talk a patient into surgery. If the surgery does not go as well as the patient has been led to expect, he will be disappointed and perhaps angry, and the surgeon's reputation will be tarnished.

Check to see that your physician is on the staff of a properly accredited hospital. If the hospital is in a major medical center, you can usually be quite certain that his credentials are above reproach. Affiliation with a hospital or medical center that is involved in research or teaching and associated with a medical school is a good indication that you are in the hands of someone reliable.

Be wary of asking a specialist in one field to recommend a specialist in another. He may suggest his golf-playing buddy, who may or may not be skillful in the extremely technical procedure you need. When choosing a surgeon, sparkling personality and bedside manner are secondary. You want the physician who is an effective technician and the best surgeon for the particular treatment you need performed.

Another word of advice. If you are contemplating surgery, do not be afraid to obtain second or even third opinions. Spinal surgery performed by a skilled technician can cure or alleviate pain from certain kinds of back disorders. However, surgery in the delicate area of the spine should never be undertaken lightly. Always make sure it is necessary by getting at least a second opinion, preferably from a surgeon of comparable training. For instance, do not see an orthopaedic surgeon who is a specialist in spinal problems, and then ask a general practitioner or general orthopaedist for a second opinion. See another orthopaedic surgeon who specializes in spinal problems.

Be wary of advice from well-meaning friends; it can be extremely frightening and totally wrong. On the other hand, the opinions of nurses, residents, and doctors who work in a hospital can be valuable. Ask them who the best technician is for the particular procedure you must undergo. At the New York Orthopaedic Hospital of the Columbia-Presbyterian Medical

Center there are twenty-one orthopaedic surgeons on the staff. Of these men, two of them exclusively do hand surgery; two mainly shoulder surgery; and two, a colleague and myself, do only spine surgery. Other orthopaedists here have sub-specialized in joint replacement or in the field of trauma. Even though we are all orthopaedic surgeons, we each have our own particular field of expertise. It would be foolhardy for a patient to come to me for hand surgery. Although I was trained in hand surgery, I have not done it for many years. Similarly, it would be ill-advised to ask a knee specialist for an opinion on spine surgery, and foolish to have him perform the operation.

It takes some time to select a physician properly, but the time spent is worth every minute. Remember, it is *your* body and you have every right to demand the best technical care available.

Seven
WHAT TO EXPECT FROM YOUR VISIT TO THE DOCTOR

Most people with backaches tend to postpone seeking professional care. Some attempt at self-diagnosis and self-help is usually warranted because a great percentage of back problems resolve by themselves with the routine treatments outlined in previous chapters. However, many people continue to delay consulting a doctor long after home measures have failed. Some simply learn, often unnecessarily, to live with daily pain. Others are afraid of what the doctor might tell them; they have severe cancer-phobia. Most of the time such concerns are unwarranted. Ninety-nine percent of all back pain is unrelated to cancer or any other such serious illness. Most backaches are a result of muscular strain in a suddenly overactive, out-of-shape person who is under stress.

If your backache does not respond to simple treatment within a week or so, or you are experiencing back pain increasingly more frequent and the pain is lasting longer, you should see a doctor. Some symptoms require immediate attention. If your back pain is accompanied by fever, difficulty in urinating or moving your bowels, numbness or tingling in either your arms or your legs, or muscle weakness and inability to properly move your fingers and toes, you should see a doctor immediately. In general, you should consult your family physician first. He will almost always be able to refer you to a specialist with whom he has had previous contact and who he knows is ethical and competent to treat back pain.

THE MEDICAL EXAMINATION

Complete History

Most doctors who specialize in back ailments really want to help you solve your problem, but they cannot succeed unless you cooperate fully. Be frank; tell your doctor *all* your symptoms and try to give them in clear historical order. Some patients are nervous or so unsettled by their symptoms that they fail to give the doctor a proper history. The history should include the past medical record as well as the chronological sequence of events leading up to the present disorder. A doctor is, after all, just like a detective trying to solve a mystery. He must know all the facts if he is to find a solution.

The doctor will take note of your symptoms and your past history and put these facts together with the clues he finds during the physical examination (called findings). He may then order certain laboratory tests before he makes his diagnosis and begins treatment. Unless you cooperate completely and tell him even what may seem to you to be relatively unimportant facts, he will not be able to give you the best possible medical care. People with backaches who more or less challenge a physician to find out what is wrong with them without giving a complete background often turn out to be malingerers or have some type of secondary gain such as a compensation payment or a court settlement in mind. In general, people who are self-employed and will lose money as a result of their inactivity tend to provide the physician with all the information possible—they are as anxious to get well as the doctor is to help them get well.

The history is the most important part of a medical examination. Before you arrive at the physician's office, jot down on a slip of paper some of your past medical history. An accurate record of your past illnesses and injuries, dating back to early childhood, can be of great value to your doctor. It is important to tell him of any severe injury or trauma, such as a fall from a tree or a motor vehicle accident. Sometimes a history of a severe infectious disease or a bout with polio could be significant. A record of past operations is also very helpful. Sometimes surgery that is not directly associated with the spine can cause adhesion formation or other complications that refer pain to the spine. Also, a history of significant medical conditions in your family for the past one or two generations can be very helpful. Many disorders have a hereditary component. Some families actually have a history of weak backs. A good example is spondylolisthesis, a slipping of either the fourth or the fifth lumbar vertebra on the vertebra or sacrum below it. This condition is transmitted genetically. Other conditions such as arthritis are also known to be familial.

It is also very important to tell your doctor what medications you have taken in the past and what drugs you are currently taking for pain relief. Some patients are reluctant to be honest about medications because they are afraid the doctor will either admonish them for taking large doses or take the medications away. Remember, you must place your trust in your doctor if you want to get proper treatment and total satisfaction from your visit. Also be certain to tell your doctor about personal habits such as alcohol intake and smoking.

Outpatient Examination

The second most important part of your visit to the doctor is the physical examination (Fig. 7–1). In general, your doctor will examine you in his office as an outpatient. He may wish to observe you as you undress. As mentioned previously, I usually prefer to see how the patient removes the shoes and steps out of his or her garments. The way in which a patient guards against spinal motions while undressing and the way he undresses will sometimes indicate exactly where the major area of muscle spasm is. Observing the patient undressing also helps identify malingering. Malingerers often shed their clothes with a certain degree of ease and then pretend that they are severely disabled and limited in all motions during the physical examination. The obvious incongruity can be a great help in determining the final diagnosis.

Usually I ask the patient to remove outer clothing. Undergarments may be left on; however, shoes and socks must be removed so that the feet can be examined. The patient then puts on an examination gown that closes in the back.

After the patient is dressed in the examination gown, I ask him to walk on his tiptoes and then on his heels so that I can evaluate limitation of motion and muscle strength in the lower

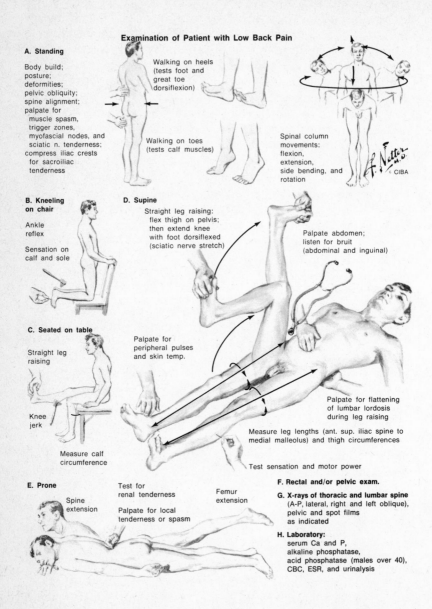

Examination of Patient with Low Back Pain

A. Standing

Body build;
posture;
deformities;
pelvic obliquity;
spine alignment;
palpate for
  muscle spasm,
  trigger zones,
  myofascial nodes, and
  sciatic n. tenderness;
compress iliac crests
  for sacroiliac
  tenderness

Walking on heels
(tests foot and
great toe
dorsiflexion)

Walking on toes
(tests calf muscles)

Spinal column
movements:
flexion,
extension,
side bending, and
rotation

B. Kneeling on chair

Ankle
reflex

Sensation on
calf and sole

D. Supine

Straight leg raising:
flex thigh on pelvis;
then extend knee
with foot dorsiflexed
(sciatic nerve stretch)

Palpate abdomen;
listen for bruit
(abdominal and inguinal)

C. Seated on table

Straight leg
raising

Knee
jerk

Palpate for
peripheral pulses
and skin temp.

Measure calf
circumference

Palpate for flattening
of lumbar lordosis
during leg raising

Measure leg lengths (ant. sup. iliac spine to
medial malleolus) and thigh circumferences

Test sensation and motor power

E. Prone

Spine
extension

Test for
renal tenderness

Palpate for local
tenderness or spasm

Femur
extension

F. Rectal and/or pelvic exam.

G. X-rays of thoracic and lumbar spine
(A-P, lateral, right and left oblique),
pelvic and spot films
as indicated

H. Laboratory:
serum Ca and P,
alkaline phosphatase,
acid phosphatase (males over 40),
CBC, ESR, and urinalysis

Figure 7–1. The examination of the patient with low back pain. (Copyright © 1980, CIBA Pharmaceutical Company)

extremities. A person who can walk well on his toes and heels has fairly normal nerve function in the lower extremities. However, if there is nerve involvement on one side, the affected leg will be markedly weaker than the opposite extremity. Next I ask the patient to kneel in a chair; holding onto the back. I then test the ankle reflexes with the use of a reflex hammer. A diminished ankle or knee reflex can be an indication of spinal nerve compression. Comparison of reflexes from one side to the other is most helpful. I then ask the patient to sit on the examining table with the knees hanging over the side. Using the reflex hammer, I check the knee reflexes. Then I measure the calves and thighs to see if they are equal. Long-standing nerve-root problems will often result in muscular wasting, causing the circumference of the calf and thigh of one leg to be smaller than those of the other.

For the next part of the examination, the patient lies on his back on the examining table. First I measure leg lengths from the pelvis and the belly button to the bony prominence on the inside of the ankle. In this way I can determine if an apparent discrepancy in length between the legs is actual or if the pelvis is higher on one side, making it appear as though one leg is shorter than the other. An apparent leg length discrepancy can be the result of a muscle spasm that causes the pelvis to be held higher on the affected side. Apparent leg length discrepancies are seen very frequently in cases of acute or chronic muscle spasm and also in scoliosis.

Minor leg length discrepancy is normal and is seen in almost everyone. In right-handed people, the right leg is longer; in left-handed people, the left leg is longer. Differences of as much as three-eighths to one-half inch are considered quite normal. Most patients I have examined with this type of leg length discrepancy have no back pain whatsoever. In fact, even after the great polio epidemic, which created many leg length differences as a result of shortening of an extremity related to the disease, the majority of patients affected did not develop back pain as they grew older. This fact and my own observations have led me to believe that adding minor lifts to one shoe to compensate for a discrepancy is generally inappropriate and of little therapeutic value.

While the patient is lying down, I will also examine the muscles of the legs and feet. First I have the patient pull up the toes and resist my pull. Also, I will ask them to push down the foot so that I can see if the calf muscles are weak. Having the patient resist while I bend the knee and straighten it out again tests calf and thigh muscle strength. Next I test each leg for a complete range of hip motion by flexing the leg at the hip with the knee bent. The opposite leg remains straight. While the leg is in this position, I try to straighten it at the knee. This test is called the straight-leg-raising test. It detects sciatic nerve irritation caused by pressure inside the spine. For example, disc herniation will often cause marked limitation of the ability to perform a straight-leg raising on the affected side. A herniated disc involving nerve roots on one side may also cause a marked impairment in straight-leg raising in the opposite leg, and this finding is also very helpful in making the proper diagnosis.

Examining hip motion will also help determine if arthritis is present in the hip joints. Arthritis of the hip can lead to severe low back pain. I have seen quite a few patients with this type of problem.

While the patient is on his back, I usually feel for the arterial pulses at the groin, in back of the knees, and at the ankles. These pulses are taken in the same way the pulse is taken at the wrist. They are especially important in elderly patients who may show diminished or even absent pulses on one side as a result of hardening of the arteries. I also feel for pulsation in the abdomen. Abnormal pulsation that can be felt during the examination is a sign of an aortic aneurysm (blowout or bulge of the largest artery of the body). The aneurysm can also be heard through the abdomen with a stethoscope.

The next part of the examination is done with the patient standing. Range of motion is tested by having the patient bend forward carefully and then to both the right and left sides. This test shows the extent of muscle spasm and causes a marked aggravation of symptoms in patients with spinal stenosis, especially in the legs and feet. When these patients arch their backs completely, curving the spine backward in what we call hyperextension, lower extremity symptoms are reproduced exactly. If these symptoms are relieved immediately when the patient bends forward in a crouching position, the diagnosis of spinal stenosis is almost certain.

At the conclusion of the exam, I will do a rectal examination in some cases. It is not usually warranted for young patients unless they have given a history of rectal bleeding or irregular bowel movements. But in adult patients, especially in males, the rectal exam is helpful because diseases of the prostate gland are very common in men and often lead to low back symptoms.

When the physical exam is finished, the patient gets dressed and returns to the consultation office to review findings and X rays and to discuss further testing. In most cases my patients have already had a thorough X-ray examination of the lower spine before they come for the physical exam. A complete series includes a film taken from back to front while the patient is standing and a side view to show the degree of swayback or lordosis. In addition, right and left oblique views of the lower spine are taken to see if any abnormality exists in the structure of the vertebrae themselves and to detect spondylolysis or spondylolisthesis. The X rays are carefully reviewed for evidence of bony abnormalities which may be congenital (present at birth) or acquired (arising after birth). In addition, evidence of old fractures as well as destruction caused by tumors can usually be identified.

After examining the X rays, I usually order a screening exam of routine chemical tests of both the urine and blood. In some patients more sophisticated tests are ordered, such as a protein screening. It is done by a system called electrophoresis and is performed to rule out some tumors and arthritic conditions.

If a condition such as spinal stenosis, a herniated disc, or a tumor is suspected, a computerized tomographic X-ray scan, called a CT scan (or CAT scan) is needed. This test usually can be done on an outpatient basis. It need not be done at the initial visit.

The CT scanner is a marvelous invention developed in the last five years as a result of research done in this country and in Europe. The computerized scanner uses a form of extremely low-dose X rays to penetrate the body. The scanner can be used to detect abnormalities in various parts of the body, including the skeleton and the internal organs. It is particularly helpful in diagnosing disorders in the brain and spine because these areas are so hard to examine by any other means.

The computerized scan allows us to examine the brain as we might examine a loaf of bread that has already been sliced. You can take a slice from the middle of the loaf and look at it from front to back and from side to side without actually injuring the loaf of bread in any way. With a computerized axial tomogram, we can examine slices from a limb, the spinal canal, or the brain on a television screen. The slice can also be magnified many times to give us a clear picture of what is going on inside the head or the spine. Technologic advances are frequent; almost every four or five months new and better computerized scanners are developed. The CT scan is particularly helpful in diagnosing spinal stenosis and for diagnosing and localizing spinal tumors and herniated discs.

If I suspect a herniated disc or some other type of intraspinal problem, I will also arrange for an electrical diagnostic study called an electromyographic examination, or EMG. For this test very fine needles are inserted into certain muscle groups in the upper and lower extremities. The electrical impulses given off by the muscles are recorded on a graph. The test records both normal and abnormal impulses and is quite sensitive when performed by an experienced technician. The results from the EMG will often clinch the final diagnosis.

Nerve-conduction studies are usually done in conjunction with an EMG. In the nerve-conduction test a certain area of a major nerve is stimulated, and the time it takes for that nerve to conduct an impulse to the muscle being examined is recorded in milliseconds. Normal nerve-conduction rates for all nerves and all muscle groups in the body have been carefully mapped out in the past by researchers. Tests are done in both the arms and the legs so that rates on one side can be compared with those on the other. This test will often help determine a specific diagnosis.

Occasionally, a skeletal problem resulting from either infection or tumor is suspected. The problem can be identified by introducing a radioisotope (a radioactive chemical element) into the body. The radioisotope attaches itself to bone and "lights up" the bone on a scan. The best form of bone scan at present is a technetium scan, in which the bone-seeking isotope is technetium methylenediphosphonate (^{99}Te-MPD). This isotope has a half-life of six hours. (The half-life is the time in which the radioactivity will be reduced by one half through radioactive decay.) The isotope is given intravenously and three hours later a special camera is used to view the spine, pelvis, and ribs. Any abnormal uptake of the isotope in these bony structures will be seen as a hot spot and help localize a problem, leading to the proper diagnosis. The test is completely painless and most helpful. It can be done in some medical centers and hospitals as an outpatient procedure.

With the findings from a complete examination of the patient and the results from the tests ordered, most disorders can be diagnosed accurately. As I've mentioned before, approximately 90 percent of all patients that I see have uncomplicated acute muscle spasm and low back pain resulting from long-term stress, improper diet, and lack of exercise. Patients with this type of back pain can be helped relatively easily and can avoid future episodes of back pain by altering their life-styles. If they are willing to control the amount of stress in their lives, cut down on improper foods and supplement their diets with proper additives, and begin routine exercise programs, most need never suffer from back pain again. However, those patients who refuse to change and who continue to do the same things that have led to back pain in the first place are likely to have recurrent episodes of backache.

Inpatient Examination

Sometimes examinations must be done in the hospital in order to come up with a proper diagnosis. Usually an in-hospital exam is necessary when the problem is more complicated and the testing equipment needed to pinpoint the problem is not available on an outpatient basis.

The *spinal tap* is an in-hospital procedure. A very narrow needle is inserted directly into one of the lower areas of the spine, and the fluid that normally flows around the spinal cord and nerve roots is then withdrawn and examined. A spinal tap is a relatively painless and easy procedure when performed by a physician who is well-trained and experienced. It is usually done under local anesthesia and takes no longer than fifteen or twenty minutes. After the test, it is important to stay flat in bed for approximately twenty-four hours. This allows the small hole made by the needle in the covering of the spinal canal to heal by itself. A standing posture prevents closure. In addition, some very few patients experience severe headaches because of persistent leakage of the spinal fluid through the small needle puncture. Remaining flat in bed will diminish the severity of these headaches tremendously.

A *myelogram* is nothing more than a spinal tap during which either air or a chemical dye is injected directly into the spinal canal. X-ray techniques are then used to see if the dye flows up and down the spinal canal properly as the patient is put in various positions. This is always done in an X-ray department, and in almost all instances spinal fluid will be taken at the same time and examined as in a spinal tap. There is a tremendous amount of fear and concern about myelograms and their effect. In the past some myelograms were done by inexperienced, poorly trained people. At Columbia-Presbyterian Medical Center we do between twenty and thirty myelograms every day and complications are extremely rare. Most patients experience little pain or discomfort.

It takes approximately forty minutes to do a myelogram. It is usually done in the neurologic X-ray department. The patient is placed on an X-ray table, which can tilt both up and down. The patient is usually in the face-down position after the myelogram dye is inserted. The lights in the room are then turned out so that the doctors can see clearly exactly what is happening inside the spinal canal. Any type of obstruction—for example, a herniated disc—will be seen on the television screen while the procedure is being done. If any abnormality is noted, a series of X-ray films is taken while the test proceeds, to give a permanent record that can be reviewed at a later date.

A myelogram is an extremely important test. In many cases it shows us conditions going on inside the spinal canal that we would be unable to detect by any other means. As mentioned before, it is not a dangerous test when done by an experienced technician, and should not be a cause for concern. After a myelogram, the patient must be confined completely in bed for twenty-four hours in the semisitting position.

Another examination that is done on an inpatient basis is the *venogram*. In this test the veins around the vertebrae are injected with a dye. The dye usually fills the blood vessels that travel around the vertebrae and the vessels around the disc area in the spine and shows any deviations from normal. A venogram can be most helpful in diagnosing a problem that myelograms and CT scans have not been able to delineate clearly.

Sometimes it is also necessary to do tests in other areas of the body to find the source of back pain. Kidney problems can cause backache, and thus an IVP—intravenous pyelogram—may sometimes be necessary. For an IVP, a dye is injected through a vein in the arm. The dye outlines the pattern of urine flow throughout the kidneys; the inside of the kidneys where the urine collects and little tubes that lead from the kidneys to the bladder can be seen clearly so that any type of obstruction or problem is obvious. Other specific tests, such as X rays of the pelvis to detect arthritis of the hips, may also be needed to clinch the diagnosis.

While the patient is in the hospital for testing, a *trial of pelvic traction* will often be done. A harness is placed around the lower portion of the spine and the patient is put in traction to diminish muscle spasm and relieve pain. Traction itself is not believed to be of any major beneficial effect; however, *it does enforce complete bed rest*. I have had hundreds of patients for whom I have prescribed *total* bed rest who have ignored my directions. Usually they call back several days or weeks later and tell me that their back pain has not improved. When I ask if they have stayed in bed, they will almost always say yes. However, if I question either their spouse or some other relative who lives with them, I learn that the patient did the wash, mowed the lawn, or engaged in some other strenuous activity! When I get this type of person into the hospital, I will often put them to bed, sedate them, and apply pelvic traction to ensure absolute bed rest. He is only allowed to leave his bed to use a bedside commode for bowel movements. This strict regimen usually results in a reduction of symptoms within two or three days. If symptoms increase, conditions other than simple muscle spasm are likely and the diagnosis can be made by the use of the specialized tests described.

Your Time to Question Your Doctor

After I give the patient the diagnosis, I discuss treatment in great detail. This is the time when the patient should present a list of questions. Any good physician will be more than happy to answer them. Never feel that your questions are stupid or unimportant. You have an absolute right to ask them, and no doctor should be too busy to answer them or make you feel embarrassed or belittled.

Sometimes questions will come to mind after you have left the doctor's office. Jot them down on a piece of paper and phone your doctor in a few days and ask him to explain anything that puzzles or alarms you. Also feel free to ask about his recommendations for treatment.

Do not be afraid to ask your doctor to call in a consultant if your problem is extremely complicated and he is not able to make the diagnosis for you. There is nothing wrong with asking for second or even third opinions, especially when an operation has been recommended. An ethical doctor is never embarrassed when a patient requests another opinion.

Family members should also feel free to ask questions. A well-informed patient and family are the greatest assets in a good treatment program. I never hesitate to have a family conference to answer relatives' questions and to allay their anxiety.

If your doctor has recommended a specific surgical procedure, there is nothing wrong with asking him about the operation that he is planning. Sometimes you can look up the specific procedures or operations he has mentioned in the medical literature. However, for some it is not always a good idea to read too much because a little knowledge can be a dangerous thing. Nonetheless, it is your right to find out everything you can about your condition, and certainly no ethical person will object to your doing so.

Eight

TREATMENT FOR ACUTE BACK PROBLEMS

The success of treatment for a painful back depends on the knowledge and experience of the doctor, as well as on the degree of patient cooperation. *Acute back pain* (severe pain and spasm occurring for the first or second time), which is discussed here, is treated differently than *chronic back pain* (pain that recurs repeatedly), which is dealt with in Chapter 9.

ABSOLUTE BED REST

The first and most important treatment for acute back pain is *absolute bed rest*. By absolute, I mean absolute! That means getting out of bed only to go to the bathroom. Unfortunately, many people do not understand what the word *absolute* means. It means 100 percent of the time! When some part of the body is in pain, the best treatment is to allow it to rest.

Absolute bed rest should be taken in a bed with a firm mattress. The patient should stay in a *semisitting* position. There are special mechanical beds available that can be positioned to support the semisitting posture, almost like a hospital bed. If you don't have the luxury of this type of bed, you can use pillows to achieve the same end. Prop several in back of your spine and put a couple underneath your knees to keep your knees bent. This posture is the most comfortable for most people. Within days, the muscle spasm should subside.

125

Remember to get up only to go to the bathroom. Meals can be taken in bed and if you absolutely have to do work, limit yourself to using the phone. Obviously, it is best to divorce yourself from *all* stressful situations and to avoid telephone calls and anything but emergency messages. Treat yourself as if you had a major surgical procedure and were incommunicado for a few days. Most of us do not take back ailments seriously enough; we try to continue working as well as keeping on top of stressful home and office situations that may have contributed greatly to the episode of back pain in the first place.

After the first couple of days of *absolute* rest, you may get out of bed to take a twenty-minute tub bath two or three times a day. Use warm, *not hot*, water. Tub baths should be taken for no longer than twenty or thirty minutes. It is important to be very careful with warm water and heating pads. I have seen patients with very severe burns on their backs and legs as a result of soaking in water so hot they could barely stand it. Some patients who have neurologic problems or diabetes actually do not feel temperature as acutely as others and can severely scald themselves. Heating pads are also dangerous, particularly if you fall asleep on one. Always wrap a heating pad in a thick towel and use only the low setting. Let someone else know you are using a heating pad so they can wake you if you fall asleep. Some patients have suffered from severe burns as well as electrical shocks when perspiring after falling asleep on a heating pad.

A regimen of tub baths, absolute bed rest, muscle relaxants (if prescribed by your doctor), and eliminating stress will usually cure back pain. However, if this program does not work in the home, then you will have to go into the hospital, where your doctor will probably put you into traction.

TRACTION

As mentioned in a previous chapter, traction's main beneficial effect is to enforce absolute bed rest. Large doses of muscle relaxants and tranquilizing drugs are given at the same time to try to free the patient from anxieties that may have aggravated the muscle spasm.

PHYSICAL MODALITIES

After the patient is placed in traction, we usually will start some form of physical treatment. These treatments are called physical modalities.

Diathermy and Massage

Diathermy is a form of shortwave radio therapy. The radio waves penetrate the skin to a depth of one to two centimeters, heating and thus soothing the muscles that are in spasm. When coupled with gentle massage by a skilled physical therapist, it can be of tremendous help. However, when back pain is severe, diathermy can sometimes make things even worse. It is usually better to wait for a day or two until the most severe pain has abated before starting.

Sometimes the best treatment for a muscular strain is an aggressive massage, administered shortly after the injury. This type of massage can be used quite effectively along with heat (sometimes alternated with ice packs) to help soothe muscle spasm. However, for severe, acute sprains, ice massage and absolute bed rest are the treatment of choice for the first day or two. After this initial period, heat treatments and massage are used to help the blood vessels draw inflammatory agents away from the injured area, and thus decrease the pain.

Ultrasound Treatments

Ultrasound treatments use high-frequency sound waves, which are usually transmitted to the patient through a fluid medium such as mineral oil. The therapist applies the conducting medium to the painful area and then moves a wand-type instrument over it. The wand transmits sound waves through the liquid medium to the inflamed muscles. The sound waves penetrate deeper than diathermy and usually go four to six centimeters into the body. Ultrasound treatments are quite safe and may be repeated over a period of three or four weeks to relieve muscle spasm. Massage is usually used in combination with diathermy, but can also be combined with ultrasound to help relieve muscle spasm. Some of the finest athletic trainers in the world use either diathermy or ultrasound coupled with massage to work out sprains and muscle spasms.

Nerve Blocks

Nerve blocks are generally anesthetic agents injected directly into a nerve center to block the pain transmission along the path of that nerve. Usually, drugs such as Xylocaine or Carbocaine are used and are given in greatly diluted concentrations so the dosage is not toxic. Nerve blocks can be used to relieve pain in many areas. They are a most effective treatment, especially when coupled with gentle massage. Sometimes the best treatment is to block a nerve in the area of muscle spasm or sprain, and then when the anesthetic has taken effect, begin a gentle massage. This regimen can break the pain cycle and is used by athletes with severe strains. It allows them to return to action within a relatively short period of time without serious injury or chronic disability.

Trigger-Point Treatments

The finest physiatrists and athletic trainers in the country have used pain trigger-point treatments for years. Areas that serve as triggers of pain can either be injected with anesthetic drugs like those mentioned in the discussion of nerve blocks, or sprayed with ethyl chloride sprays. Both treatments can be tremendously effective. Remarkable results have been obtained, especially in ballerinas and professional athletes who must get back into action quickly. Trigger points are similar to the acupuncture points blocked with needles during acupuncture.

DMSO

DMSO or dimethyl sulfoxide, a by-product of the wood pulp industry, was thought for years to be of absolutely no value. Later research revealed that DMSO could be used to treat a variety of disorders. DMSO penetrates the skin rapidly and quickly attacks inflamed and spasmed muscles. It is one of a few substances that can be absorbed through the skin into the bloodstream, and thus rapidly spreads throughout the body.

DMSO has been used most effectively to reduce pain and swelling from bursitis, tendonitis, strains, and sprains. It can also be used to clear up skin ulcers and relieve the pain of bedsores and shingles.

DMSO treatments were tremendously popular about twelve years ago. However, some studies done at that time showed that DMSO has potentially toxic effects and can cause cataracts in experimental animals. As a result, the Food and Drug Administration has not approved its use, and at present, DMSO is only available to veterinarians for use on animals.

There are a few people who continue to use DMSO illegally. Until the government gives the green light, I would consider these treatments to be unsafe and risky. Like so many other "wonder drugs," DMSO was overpublished in the media before it had been properly evaluated. Studies underway now should clarify the toxicity of DMSO within the next few years. Research should identify the impurities that cause the side effects. Once they can be removed we will have an effective drug we can use safely in recommended doses.

Cortisone Injections

About twenty-five years ago cortisone drugs were routinely injected directly into an inflamed muscle or tender joint. Since then the hazards of using cortisone, a drug that is absorbed easily into the bloodstream, have become obvious. One or two injections of a small amount of cortisone into a tender area or joint are perfectly safe. However, repeated injections can be hazardous and cause serious side effects, among them cartilage destruction in the joints.

Cortisone that is to be injected is usually mixed with a very slowly absorbed base solution and a local anesthetic agent such as Xylocaine. Treatment can give prolonged relief from acute muscle spasm or arthritic attacks. However, as with most medications and treatments, while moderate doses are helpful, too much can be harmful!

Hot and Cold Packs

Hot and cold packs are traditional treatments for backaches and are extremely effective in reducing muscle spasm and pain. A hydrocollator, which is a heat-absorbing material, will provide a soothing effect for twenty or thirty minutes. Alternating applications of heat and cold at ten-minute intervals will sometimes produce astounding results. This technique has been used in health spas and clinics throughout the world. Warm mud packs, which produce a soothing heat, and mineral water baths can also be of great help. A physiatrist or therapist can usually recommend a program of proven effectiveness. A massage using ice can offer dramatic relief for acute muscle injuries and ligament sprains, especially when started before tissue swelling (edema) has fully developed.

Electrical Stimulation

The technique of electrically stimulating the nerves through the skin is referred to as transcutaneous electrical nerve stimulation, or TENS, and has been in use for the past six or seven years. An electrical device that transmits a low-wave electric pulse is used to stimulate the skin at trigger points that are known to set up pain patterns. TENS trigger points are nearly identical to acupuncture points.

Patients can wear the TENS device and stimulate trigger areas as often as necessary to relieve pain. Electrodes are taped directly over the area of greatest pain, and the patient can then stimulate this area for as little as fifteen minutes or as long as two hours repeatedly during the day. Stimulation breaks the pattern of muscle spasm that induces pain, which in turn causes increased spasm. TENS devices help the patient relieve spasm rapidly and allow the patient to resume normal motion relatively quickly.

The TENS device is powered by small, high-potency batteries. The patient can control the frequency and amplitude of the electrical impulses with small dials in the device. Some patients describe the tingling sensation experienced as pleasant. The machine is expensive, about $350, and at present the cost is not always covered by insurance.

Many patients with spinal cord injuries have been treated with TENS devices. Approximately 50 percent have reported an improvement in painful spasms. TENS therapy works particularly well for conditions such as bursitis, arthritis, and low back pain, and for best results should be used in combination with other forms of treatment such as acupuncture and massage. Recently these devices have also been used to reduce the incision pain that occurs during the first five or six days after surgery.

For severe chronic pain, a highly sophisticated type of TENS stimulator can actually be inserted surgically in the body. Neurosurgeons have perfected a technique that allows them to implant electrodes with hair-thin wires either in the spinal cord or in the brain itself. The wires lead to a small radio-activated electrical source that is placed just under the skin of the chest. To activate the device, the patient presses a radio transmitter against the chest. The device then sends tiny electrical impulses into either the brain or the spinal cord, causing targeted nerve cells to fire. The process causes release of beta-endorphin, a painkilling substance produced by the body's own nerve cells, which appears to be related to morphine. Implanted TENS devices have successfully relieved back pain and muscle spasm for periods lasting from several hours to several days in some patients. Unfortunately, others develop a tolerance to this technique after several weeks or months and then need other forms of treatment.

Hypnosis

Hypnosis can be an important form of self-help as well as a form of treatment provided by a trained therapist. Dr. Herbert Spiegel of the Columbia-Presbyterian Medical Center has been most successful in treating chronic pain syndromes with hypnosis so the patient can "turn off" pain whenever it occurs. Other psychiatrists give the patient a cassette recording of the hypnotic induction so that he can play it whenever spasm and pain occur.

Hypnosis can provide effective pain relief and help the patient resume normal activities quickly. It is a very valuable form of treatment.

Biofeedback

Biofeedback techniques teach the patient to alter body activities that are normally not under voluntary control. Levels of body activity—for example, the degree of muscle tension—are recorded and projected on a TV screen. The patient watches the projected patterns and learns how to alter them to improve health or relieve pain. With biofeedback, patients can learn to control heartbeat, muscle spasms, and many other body functions.

Doctors are always advising patients to relax, but learning to relax isn't easy. With biofeedback, however, the patient can actually see his level of tension projected on a television monitor, and then learn how to manipulate that tension and decrease it. In time, he will learn to control tension even when he is not watching the monitor. Biofeedback laboratories are now open in centers throughout the country. In addition to learning how to counteract back pain, patients can be taught to effectively fight the stresses that can cause headaches, high blood pressure, insomnia, phobias, and speech problems. Biofeedback doesn't always teach you how to eliminate your pain, but it can teach you how to live around it.

Gravity Traction

A newly introduced form of therapy, gravity traction, is really nothing new at all; it dates back to the time of Hippocrates. In those days people with backaches were strapped to ladderlike frames, turned upside down, and lowered suddenly to the ground. The jolt caused sudden stretching—a form of aggressive traction that probably had some manipulative effect on the patient's spine as well. According to the records of that era, this form of treatment was fairly effective.

A modified form of gravity traction is now being used more and more in institutions throughout the United States. The patient is strapped onto a circle-type bed, and traction is applied progressively at the pelvis. The bed is then tilted so that the patient is almost erect. The degree is slowly increased until the patient's spine is straightened and the muscle spasm decreased. The technique seems to work well for many people, but frankly, my feeling is that it works chiefly because it removes the patient from stressful situations and enforces bed rest.

Manipulation and Adjustments

Manipulation and spinal adjustment by a qualified osteopath or chiropractor can be of great value in treating certain conditions.

An example is a dislocated or subluxated facet joint. This condition causes a tremendous amount of pain and muscle spasm, which can be relieved when these areas are manipulated back into proper alignment. I do not hesitate to recommend manipulation, but do caution you to choose a practitioner who is qualified and who has considerable experience. Manipulation by an unskilled technician can cause severe aggravation of symptoms and even serious spinal nerve or spinal cord injury. I have seen patients who have suffered very serious disabilities and even permanent injury as a result of injudicious manipulation.

GRADUATED EXERCISE PROGRAM

As mentioned in the section on exercises (see Chapter 3), the five Keim Preventive Exercises (KPEs) should be done daily to avoid back pain in the first place. However, once back pain has occurred, the exercise program must begin with the six Pain-Relieving Exercises (PREs) shown in Fig. 3–12. The PREs should be undertaken gradually once the muscle spasm has subsided. Never do exercises while you have severe muscle spasm and pain; you could aggravate the condition and make it worse. However, once the muscle spasm and pain have ebbed slightly, start the six PREs. They will strengthen your spine and prevent recurrence of pain.

The most important thing to remember is to warm up gently before you start and not to try to do too much too soon. Each exercise should be repeated only three or four times for the first few days. Then you can increase the repetitions by one every two or three days, until you work up to a level appropriate for you.

WEIGHT CONTROL

Controlling your weight is one of the most important things you can do to help cure your back problems. A program of daily exercise will help tremendously with weight control. Do the PREs to help relieve pain after a back injury and begin a more strenuous program of weight control and muscle-strengthening exercises as soon as possible. If you really want to avoid back pain in the future, you must change your life-style. Once muscle spasm has gone, begin the daily KPE routine. In addition, learn to do some other type of physical activity every single day, rain or shine. It doesn't matter which activity you choose; it can be tennis, running, swimming, bowling, or just taking a daily brisk walk. The important thing to remember is to devote thirty or forty minutes a day to maintaining a healthy body. Your investment will bring you many pain-free, healthy years.

If you wish to join a health spa that specializes in weight reduction and exercise programs, consult with the personnel there, who should be able to set up an exercise program tailored to your needs. Ask your physician if he has specific recommendations or prohibitions. If there are questions, ask the spa instructor to call your doctor directly. Most devices used at spas—for example, the Nautilus exercise device, are safe for a patient with back problems if used properly.

Weight control is best achieved with exercise and calorie counting. Groups such as Overeaters Anonymous or Weight Watchers can be of great help. Educate yourself about food. Find out which foods contain the most calories and limit your intake. Find a sensible diet plan that will help you reduce and at the same time train you to eat properly. Avoid fad diets! Generally, diets that are high in protein and low in carbohydrates and fats work well if strictly adhered to. Consult your doctor before beginning any restrictive diet.

STRESS CONTROL

Stress is one of the three major causes of back pain. Although no one can totally avoid stress, most of us can learn to live with stressful situations more easily and find ways to reduce them. Stress is caused by tension and anxiety that build up either at home or at work. It affects absolutely everyone at some time or another. It can be, and usually is, a result of a culmination of small everyday anxieties and tensions; or it can follow a single precipitating catastrophe, such as the death of a loved one or an auto accident. Stress can lead to frequent emotional crises and finally a physical or mental breakdown. Physical effects often turn up in the back as severe muscle spasm and pain.

Can we avoid or at least reduce stress? Certainly! Others have done it. The most important thing is to face up to the problems we have. If you hate your job, change it—or at least try to eliminate stressful areas. If your marriage is unhappy, face the problem and try to work it out. My own solution to stress is to confront the problem directly and try to solve it. If I cannot solve it, I make a change. I have found that there is almost always a socially acceptable, mature, sensible way to solve a problem.

CORSETS AND BRACES

Although corsets and braces can be a great help during a period of acute back pain, they can become addictive. Corsets and braces reduce spinal motion, and thus reduce muscle spasm. However, they should be used only for *short periods of time*, usually no more than three or four weeks, or muscle weakness will occur. The corset used for back pain is a surgical-type garment with metal stays. It is worn during active periods and need not be worn in bed. Corsets are often used to reduce pain while driving.

Braces are even more addictive than corsets, because braces immobilize the spine to a much greater degree. If a brace is worn for four or five months, muscle atrophy and wasting will occur. Braces are used after fractures of the spine, but should be weaned from patients as rapidly as possible. Patients should learn to substitute their muscle strength instead.

It is very important not to become married to your corset or brace. Once you become dependent on such a device, it is almost impossible to go without it. You can wean yourself from the corset or brace by slowly increasing the time that you are out of it. In this way, you will gradually strengthen the muscles that God has given you to hold your spine erect and still avoid muscle spasm and backache. Couple the weaning from the corset or brace with the six PRE exercises, and eventually, when all pain and spasm go away, add the five KPE exercises.

SURGERY FOR ACUTE SPINAL PROBLEMS

Occasionally it is necessary to resort to surgery for an acute problem in the spine. Usually, surgery is necessary for the type of severely herniated disc that causes muscle or foot weakness resulting in floppiness of the foot (foot drop). Foot drop signals a neurologic problem that is advancing and getting worse. Surgery is imperative and should be done as soon as possible. Any time a neurologic problem is getting worse, surgical correction should not be delayed or it may not be possible to restore the patient to the preinjury state of health.

When surgery is recommended for an acute problem, make sure the surgeon you have selected is skilled in doing the particular technique recommended (see Chapters 6 and 7) and get a second or third opinion if you so desire. A skilled and sympathetic physician will not object to your efforts to ensure that you are getting the best possible care.

Nine

TREATMENT FOR CHRONIC BACK PROBLEMS

HOSPITAL CARE AND TRACTION

In the previous chapter we talked about treatment for acute back pain. As mentioned, the term *acute* indicates a condition that has occurred recently and for only the first or second time. The term *chronic* refers to conditions that occur repeatedly, sometimes over a period of many years. Chronic conditions tend to strike when you least expect them and usually at a time when your life is most complicated. As mentioned in previous chapters, emotional stress is an important cause of back pain. It is at a time of crisis when you are not active and are distressed emotionally that back pain is likely to strike.

In general, people who have chronic back problems have already seen a doctor on more than one occasion. Usually he has outlined a treatment program which, in most cases, will resemble that given in Chapter 8. Many patients with chronic back pain will agree to treatment that includes an exercise program with weight reduction, but then fail to follow through with the program after the initial pain subsides. They fail to understand that *they must change their life-style* if they want to have a pain-free back in the future. As the months and years go by, they continue a life-style of emotional stress, improper diet, and physical lethargy until a vicious cycle of chronic back pain develops. Many patients I see have suffered from back pain for fifteen or twenty years. They spend at least four to twelve weeks a year confined to a bed. While the pain is severe they are anxious to do anything that is necessary to relieve it, but as soon as things get better they rapidly fall back into old patterns. They go through life anticipating the next episode of chronic, incapacitating muscle spasm and pain.

In general, the care for chronic back pain is the same as for acute back pain. However, treatment for chronic back pain is more complicated because the patient has already been on medication (sometimes for many years). Frequently he must be hospitalized to enforce absolute bed rest. Often traction must be applied; either direct pelvic traction or gravity traction (page 132) may be used. Sometimes getting the patient away from his normal environment and enforcing total bed rest for a prolonged period will be all that is necessary to break the chronic pain cycle. After repeated bouts of pain, the doctor may be able to convince the patient that a major change in life-style is necessary. In general, however, most patients return to their previous way of life shortly after their backache improves.

DAILY PHYSICAL THERAPY

While hospitalized, most patients will be given diathermy or ultrasound treatments and massage. These techniques work very well if performed by a skilled physical therapist. In addition, a physiatrist may be called in to treat pain trigger points with local injections or ethyl chloride sprays (page 128). Often physical therapy in combination with a break from the everyday stressful environment will be enough to end an episode of back pain.

SURGERY

Most people have a healthy, quite normal, fear of surgery. However, if this fear becomes exaggerated, it may keep a patient from accepting a surgical treatment that could cure or relieve him of incapacitating pain. For certain specific spinal problems, surgery, if performed properly, can provide an almost miraculous cure. When the diagnosis is made correctly and the surgery performed by a skilled technician, spinal surgery will almost always provide excellent results. Only the malingerer or severely neurotic or psychotic patient will fail to be cured under these circumstances. Nonetheless, many people continue to be excessively fearful of spinal surgery.

Spinal surgery got a bad reputation twenty or thirty years ago when it was frequently attempted by poorly trained surgeons or by surgeons who lacked the necessary technical skill. This type of surgery is extremely difficult, and requires years of extra training. However, training alone is not enough. The surgeon must also have a certain degree of natural skill as well. In this sense, surgeons are like violinists. Anyone can attend music school and learn to play the violin. After eight years even those with very little talent can play many compositions. However, only those few who have a very real gift will become virtuoso performers. The same is true of people in technical fields such as surgery. A surgeon can train extensively, and even subspecialize in the field of spinal surgery for several years, and still not be a gifted technician. Certain men and women will naturally excel in technical fields like surgery that require incredible manual dexterity. Their talent is God-given and no amount of training can take its place.

How do you, the patient, find such a surgeon? Follow the guidelines given in Chapter 6, How to Choose Your Doctor. Look for a physician who has done several thousand of these operations. Finally, ask other patients. The best form of referral is usually a satisfied patient, and surgeons who specialize in one type of surgery will have hundreds of satisfied patients who are more than happy to recommend them.

There are many different spinal operations that are performed to relieve back pain. In the next section these operations will be described. In addition, I will review the hospital course, what to expect from surgery, and certain procedures that are usually performed as adjuncts to surgery.

Epidural Injections With Cortisone Drugs and Local Anesthesia

As mentioned in Chapter 8, the term *epidural* is used to refer to injection of a drug into the area just outside of the dura. The dura is the thick membrane that encases the spinal cord and related structures as well as the cerebrospinal fluid, which circulates throughout the brain and spinal canal. Cortisone-type drugs can be injected into the epidural area in the lower part of the spine, along with a local anesthetic to treat inflammatory nerve-root compression or occasionally a herniated disc. Epidural injections effectively relieve pain in these disorders but do not prevent a recurrence, especially if there is chronic nerve-root impingement as a result of spinal stenosis or arthritic changes of the facet joints.

Facet Denervation (Facet Rhizotomy)

The facets are the small joints on either side of the back of the vertebrae. These joints move slightly to allow forward bending and twisting. Specific nerves that carry pain fibers pass near to the facet joints as they leave the spine and will cause back pain if the joint compresses or impinges on them. For the last fifteen years researchers have tried to block the tiny nerve branches that encircle the facet joints by coagulating them with a high-frequency electrical current. This approach is called *facet denervation* or *facet rhizotomy and* is only effective in relieving pain that originates from the facet joints. Facet denervation has little effect on problems that are a result of conditions directly within the spinal canal. In the last five years, many experts have begun to use this technique after other nonoperative treatments—including bed rest, muscle relaxants, acupuncture, biofeedback, and exercises—have failed.

A facet rhizotomy is performed with the patient under local anesthesia and lying face down on an X-ray table. A needle of small diameter is inserted through the skin and muscles until it touches the facet to be treated. An X-ray fluoroscope is used so that the doctor can guide the needle accurately in the body. Once the needle is properly placed, an electrical current is passed through it to destroy the little nerves around the facet joints.

When facet rhizotomy was first introduced, it showed great promise for success. However, results in a large series of patients have failed to prove that the technique is predictably effective, and long-lasting cures are infrequent. Nevertheless, facet rhizotomy does not require an extensive surgical invasion of the body and is certainly quite safe. A trial with it is unlikely to cause any serious future problems and may make more invasive procedures such as surgery unnecessary. Facet denervation works successfully in certain patients and unpredictably fails miserably in others.

Microsurgery

An exciting medical technique now being used in spinal surgery is microsurgery. It allows an operation to be performed through a small incision, usually less than an inch in length, made directly to the side of the midline of the spine. A small tube is inserted under X-ray control to the appropriate area, and an arthroscope is passed through it. The arthroscope is a small device, used successfully in knee operations and in other parts of the body, that allows the surgeon to see the area in question and to perform very fine procedures there.

One of my professors, who was world-renowned in the surgical treatment of the spine, used to say "You can't fix a fine watch through a keyhole." Another of his favorite sayings was "You can't fix a fine watch in an inkwell." Both statements underscore the limitations of microsurgery in the spine. It is impossible to complete any significant surgery through this very small instrument in an area of unusually complicated anatomy, particularly when you are not viewing it directly but through the arthroscope. Also, the major blood vessels in and around the spine make it difficult to control bleeding through an arthroscope, and serious injury can occur.

Microsurgery can best be used in spinal surgery for an acute disc herniation. In this case a surgeon, working through the arthroscope, can remove the protruding portion of the disc and thus relieve the patient's sciatica. In cases of spinal stenosis, microsurgery is impractical because it would be almost impossible to remove large amounts of bone and trace the spinal nerves out of their foramina (windows). Microsurgery cannot replace *open* spinal surgery performed by a skilled technician. Its main advantages are that it is a much smaller procedure that results in minimal scarring, a marked decrease in hospitalization, and most importantly, decreased blood loss. These advantages are usually outweighed by the risk of serious complications if structures within the spinal canal are injured.

Chymopapain

Chymopapain injection is a technique developed by Dr. Lyman
Smith of Elgin, Illinois, that is currently not available in the
United States. Natives on South Sea islands tenderize their
meat by wrapping it in papaya leaves to soften the muscle fibers.
Dr. Smith reasoned that the active ingredient in the papaya leaf
could be effectively used to break down the tissues in an
intervertebral disc and therefore make disc surgery unnecessary. His concept was excellent, and it was soon learned that the
active ingredient was an enzyme called chymopapain (an ingredient found in meat tenderizers).

   The idea of injecting chymopapain into the intervertebral disc was innovative. Dr. Smith started out experimenting
on laboratory animals to see if the enzyme would dissolve the
intervertebral disc without damaging nerve roots and surrounding structures. His experiments showed that the enzyme would
dissolve disc material without injuring the nerves themselves as
long as chymopapain was not injected directly into the nerve
itself. He used chymopapain, which was made by a pharmaceutical company in Chicago, and obtained permission from
the Food and Drug Administration to run a series of experimental tests on humans. The results in most cases were dramatic
when the patients were properly selected. By selected, I mean
that not all people with back pain were suitable candidates for
chymopapain injection. Those best suited were patients with an
isolated herniated disc pressing on one or more nerve roots that
could be visualized on a myelogram or a CT scan.

   Before a chymopapain treatment is given, a discogram is
taken of the suspected herniated disc. The discogram is an X ray
taken after dye has been injected directly into the disc space.
The dye outlines the disc on the X ray. If the dye leaks through
the disc's posterior border, the disc is considered to be ruptured
and unstable, and the patient is considered to be a good
candidate for chymopapain injection. In recent years, however,
it has been demonstrated that the results of the discogram are
not reliable and that even when disc problems are accurately
shown, degenerative disc disease that is a result of aging does
not necessarily cause back pain.

   During the experimental period, chymopapain was used
in a large number of patients with excellent results in some.

However, several side effects soon appeared. Approximately one out of every five hundred patients treated were allergic to the enzyme. In fact, a few reactions were so severe that in certain hospitals the technique was discontinued.

Because of the controversy surrounding the technique, the Food and Drug Administration has investigated the matter in detail. Neurosurgeons and orthopaedic surgeons disagree about the efficacy of the technique; there are profound and convincing arguments on both sides. In an effort to solve this dispute, a double-blind study was designed by the Food and Drug Administration and carried out in several leading medical centers. (By double-blind, we mean that neither the patient nor the physician knew whether the injection given contained chymopapain or a nonreactive drug called a *placebo*.) The study showed that chymopapain was no more effective than the so-called placebo.

Unfortunately, the entire double-blind study was later declared invalid when researchers questioned whether the placebo used was actually chemically inert, as was originally thought. Some felt the placebo itself had some dissolving action on the disc material.

At the present time a triple-blind study is being carried out under the auspices of the Food and Drug Administration. Not only is chymopapain being studied, but also the placebo that was given with chymopapain in the double-blind study. A totally inert substance is now being used as the placebo. This is all very confusing, but necessary to protect you, the consumer, from possible injury.

Another potential problem with chymopapain treatments is loss of disc height. The discs are relatively thick and add considerable height to the spinal column. If all the discs were removed, a person who is five feet eight inches tall would lose almost a foot in height. Removal of the disc between two vertebrae will decrease the space between the two vertebrae the disc separated and change the anatomic relationship between them. Specifically, the facet joints at the back of the vertebrae will be disrupted, which could in time lead to nerve root entrapment and spinal stenosis (page 56 and Figs. 4–7 D and E).

As mentioned, chymopapain treatments are illegal in the United States at the present time unless performed in one of the control centers doing the triple-blind study. However, some patients go to Canada and Mexico to have this technique performed. In the hands of skilled technicians, excellent results have been reported, but serious side effects have also shown up.

Spinal Exploration

Spinal surgery is technically difficult and physically demanding. It is a challenging field. Results can be fantastic but cannot be guaranteed. As Hippocrates said, "The occasion instant ... , decision difficult."

Usually, the physical examination, laboratory tests, and other tests ordered give me a good idea of what I will find during surgery. If a myelogram and CT scan have been taken, it may pinpoint the problem exactly. Nevertheless, until the surgery is under way, I can never be absolutely sure what the problem is and what other complicating factors may be present. That is why it is important to choose a surgeon who is experienced in all types of spinal surgery.

When I do spinal surgery, I do not say I am doing a specific operation—for example, for a herniated disc—but call the operation "a spinal exploration." By exploration, I do not mean an expedition with absolutely no sense of direction—the results of the diagnostic examination and tests have told me where to look and what to look for. During surgery, I explore the problem area, nerve roots, and vertebrae to determine the exact location of the disease or problem (pathology) and then take appropriate steps to correct it.

Spinal explorations in the lower lumbar spine should involve more than one pair of vertebrae to be certain that all of the patient's spinal nerves are completely free and decompressed. I make a practice of examining the nerves as they exit from the spine at *several levels* to be sure that no form of entrapment is present. Then I know that I have identified and solved all the problems within the spine. In one patient, two or even three different problems can be at the root of back pain. If neighboring joint spaces are not explored, a second or even third problem could be missed.

To Fuse or Not to Fuse—That Is the Question! Surgery for a herniated disc is often combined with a technique known as spinal fusion. The fusion technique predates disc herniation surgery. The very first spinal fusion in the world was performed by Dr. Russell Hibbs at the New York Orthopaedic Hospital, which later became affiliated with the Columbia-Presbyterian Medical Center. Dr. Hibbs performed this operation in 1911 to treat spinal tuberculosis. It was a remarkable feat accomplished without blood replacement or antibiotics. Dr. Hibbs was a man of great vision and an outstanding technician. He was the chief officer of the New York Orthopaedic Hospital and performed many successful spinal operations until his death in 1934. Shortly after he presented his original findings (about 1915), many other physicians investigated his results. They found that welding one or more vertebrae together with bone grafts (spinal fusion) was an effective and excellent way to immobilize movable areas of the spine and relieve back pain.

The very first disc operation was performed by Drs. Mixter and Barr in Boston in 1934. Dr. Mixter was a neurosurgeon and Dr. Barr an orthopaedic surgeon. They worked together, using a team approach. They were the first to accurately describe how disc material herniates and traps the nerve root, and to demonstrate that the nerve root could be decompressed by surgically removing the offending disc and then fusing the two vertebrae it separated.

Over the next twenty years, the technique of disc excision with spine fusion became known throughout the medical world, and literally thousands of patients underwent combined disc surgery and spinal fusion. Unfortunately, many surgeons who were not as gifted as Drs. Mixter and Barr started to do this type of surgery, and many patients obtained poor end results, bringing an ill-deserved disrepute to the fusion technique in particular. Actually, spinal fusion, if properly performed, is an outstanding technique that provides excellent results.

The fusion technique has been refined since the era of Dr. Hibbs, most notably by Dr. Melvin Watson. In 1945 he developed the bilateral-lateral spine fusion technique, which greatly increased the success rate for fusion surgery. Today, a spinal fusion performed by a skilled technician using the bilateral-lateral technique and bone grafts taken directly from the patient's own pelvis has an extremely high chance of succeeding. As techniques and surgeons' skills improve, the success rate should climb even higher (Fig. 9–1).

In general, spinal fusion should be performed if one or more of the following situations (known as indications) is

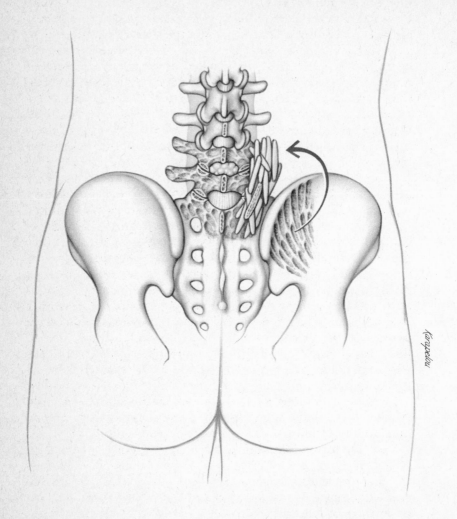

Figure 9–1. Spinal fusion technique. A bone graft is taken from the pelvic bone, usually on the right side, and placed along the prepared vertebrae at the lower portion of the spine to weld them together. This fusion takes approximately six months for the bones to become solid. During that time the spine must be protected, usually in a lumbar corset. (© Columbia University, 1981)

present: (1) X-ray evidence of unstable joints in the spine, (2) a bony defect such as spondylolysis or spondylolisthesis that is painful or growing progressively worse, (3) congenital abnormalities such as a transitional vertebra (page 77), (4) spinal instability as evidenced by a long history of low back pain that preexists new symptoms related to a specific disc herniation, (5) instability found at the time of surgery (when an unusual range of vertebral motion may be noted), if no disc herniation or other pathology is found, (6) facet instability that is noted during surgery after a tumor that has invaded the facet joints is removed, (7) generalized arthritic changes or spondylolysis at *one* level, (8) a back disorder requiring surgery in a person who regularly puts unusual stress on his spine—for example, a manual laborer or athlete, and (9) disc disease or pathology that is found in more than one level of the spine, for example between both the fourth and fifth lumbar vertebrae and the sacrum. (When more than one disc is affected, disc degeneration is probably a result of instability and a fusion is thus indicated.) Finally, spinal fusion is indicated in patients with back pain who have had previous spinal surgery that didn't include a fusion. Most of these patients have marked degenerative spinal changes that are a result of the previous operation, and a solid fusion will enhance the results of the current corrective procedure.

Just as there are indications for surgery, there are also what we call contraindications to surgery. Spinal fusion is not indicated as an adjunct to disc excision or nerve root decompression in the following situations: (1) in acute disc herniation at one level only, without any facet or joint arthritic damage, (2) in a very young person with an isolated disc herniation, (3) in people sixty or older whose spines are rigid and stable or who have generalized arthritic changes throughout the entire spine, (4) in patients with a weak heart, high blood pressure, or other conditions that would increase the operative risk, (5) in degenerative disease or spondylosis that affects more than one level of the spine—greater stress leading to back pain will occur at the vertebrae above and below the fusion, and (6) in the presence of infection with the exception of those infections like spinal tuberculosis where fusion is the recommended treatment. Finally, fusion is not recommended for those with psychiatric problems. Their postoperative course would be complicated if surgery were prolonged to include a fusion, and these patients usually recover faster when as little surgery as possible is performed.

It is best to let your surgeon decide whether fusion is necessary in your own particular case. A man skilled in spinal exploration and fusion who feels that a fusion is indicated should be allowed to proceed. In his hands, fusion will probably be the best technique for you. However, if the surgeon is not skilled in spinal fusion techniques and does not recommend it, then you would be best off with a simple disc excision or nerve root decompression.

The final word is not in on this controversy. I fear that many patients who are treated now with microsurgery or chymopapain injections will eventually develop spinal nerve entrapment syndromes or spinal stenosis, especially with age. Many of these people will then need a second or even a third operation to stabilize their spines.

My own belief is that in certain cases spinal fusion is absolutely necessary and even mandatory, and in other situations it is not indicated at all. If you have confidence in your surgeon and know that he has an excellent reputation in spinal surgery, then you should allow him to make the final decisions. Do not tie his hands by extracting a preoperative promise to either fuse or not fuse, because his decision often depends on what he finds at surgery.

Whether your surgery is best performed by an orthopaedic surgeon or a neurosurgeon depends strictly on the training that particular surgeon has had. In most Eastern medical schools, neurosurgeons do most of the nerve root decompressions; however, in the Midwestern and Western medical schools orthopaedic surgeons do a great percentage of disc surgery. Therefore, the type of specialist you choose is less important than whether the surgeon chosen has the experience in doing the technique indicated in your case.

Recovery after a simple spinal decompression is faster than after a combined fusion-decompression procedure. Patients are usually out of the hospital eight to ten days after decompressive surgery, and are usually up and about on their second or third day after the operation. Although it is best to get patients moving as early as possible to prevent complications such as clots in the veins of the legs, the two- or three-day rest is necessary because movement is quite painful and difficult for the patient at first. This rest period also allows the patient time to recover from the effects of the anesthetic. Patients who have had a spinal fusion with nerve root decompression will usually require three or four days of bed rest and cannot leave the hospital until the tenth or eleventh day.

After a spinal fusion the patient must avoid heavy lifting and twisting motions for a period of five to six months. Most fusion patients wear a soft corset, not to immobilize their spine, but to remind them to be careful. I have had many patients who feel so good two or three months after their surgery that they start doing stupid things like wrestling or playing aggressive sports. They forget that their spinal fusion is not yet mature and needs further protection until it is completely solid.

Surgery for a Herniated Disc Many of the principles outlined in the previous chapters apply to surgery for a herniated disc (the nucleus pulposus). I usually approach the disc by removing bone from the posterior portion of the vertebrae directly over the area where preoperative tests have indicated the problem. After removing the disc herniation at this level I explore either one or two additional disc spaces to be certain that they are properly decompressed and that no problem is present there. I trace the nerve roots and follow them as they leave the spinal canal through their individual foramina. If a nerve root decompression is indicated, it can usually be done without difficulty. Spinal fusion can be combined with disc excision if indicated (Fig. 9–2).

Surgery for Spinal Stenosis As has been mentioned previously (page 56) spinal stenosis is a condition caused by arthritic changes in the posterior joints (facets) and spondylosis, (other degenerative change), in the disc joint. The usually triangular spinal canal becomes narrowed both from front to back and from side to side. Narrowing of the canal causes pinching or entrapment of the nerve roots. Spinal stenosis can be diagnosed by a myelogram and CT scan. The entrapped nerves must be decompressed and freed; the nerve roots must be traced out of the spinal canal to ensure that all segments of the nerve are free. In most instances, decompression must be carried out at more than one spinal level. The procedure is long and arduous; and in younger patients, a spinal fusion must be done as well to add stability to the spine. In people over the age

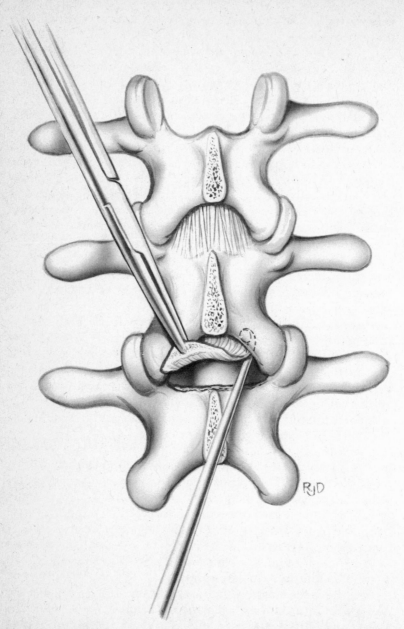

Figure 9–2A. Illustration of the approach to a lower lumbar disc region. The ligament between the vertebrae is first excised so that the spinal contents can be exposed.

of sixty, spinal fusions are rarely needed because the vertebrae become more stable with increasing age.

Spinal stenosis is being diagnosed more and more frequently. It is especially common in patients who have had disc excisions without spinal fusions. Later, the remnant of the disc is lost through degeneration and the vertebrae above and below the affected disc space come closer together, causing nerve root entrapment (Figs. 9–3 and 9–4).

Surgery for Spondylolisthesis Spondylolysis and spondylolisthesis are conditions for which there is a genetic predisposition that is triggered by repeated stress or trauma. These conditions are rare before age five, but are often seen between ages five and twenty, at which time they tend to progress. In adults, spondylolisthesis is a stable condition that rarely progresses. It may, however, be complicated by a herniated disc.

Surgery for spondylolisthesis (slipping of one vertebral body on the body below it) consists of decompressing the nerve roots, which have been stretched and kinked by the slipped vertebrae and the bony deposits that occur at that level. It is quite difficult to reposition the vertebra once it has slipped, so in most cases the vertebrae are fused in the position in which they are at the time of surgery. In rare instances, usually in young children, the vertebra can actually be repositioned correctly. If nerve root impingement is noted during the operation, the nerves must be adequately decompressed or the patient will not be relieved of sciatica and hamstring-muscle spasm.

Surgery for Tumors Fortunately, most tumors in the spine are benign (not cancerous). These tumors grow very slowly and eventually cause direct pressure on nerve roots, leading to severe pain in the lower extremities along the course of the sciatic nerve. In most instances, an exact diagnosis can be made before surgery by a CT scan and/or a myelogram. Usually, after the excision of a tumor, the spinal elements are found to be unstable and a bilateral-lateral spinal fusion must be performed. Occasionally, tumors are found in the body or the posterior elements of the vertebrae.

On rare occasions, malignant tumors are found in the spinal area. If these can be diagnosed beforehand by the use of biopsy, surgery can often be avoided, and X-ray therapy can be used instead. If the malignant tumor involves only one vertebra, the entire vertebra can occasionally be excised. This procedure

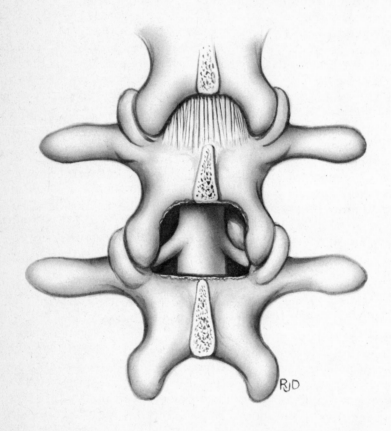

Figure 9–3. This illustration shows a herniated disc pressing on the nerve root on the right side. Once the disc is removed and the nerve root is free of its pressure, the pain going down the leg will be relieved.

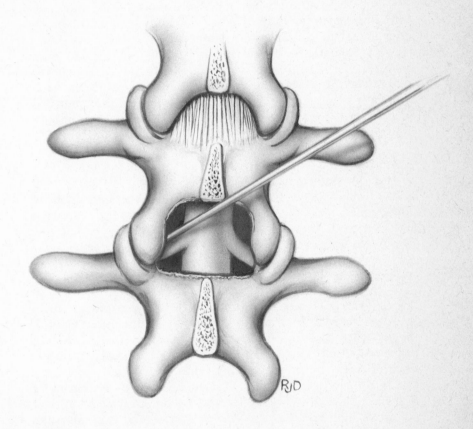

Figure 9–4. This figure illustrates the nerve roots already freed of any entrapment. The canal where the nerve roots exit is then probed to be certain that there are no further bony or disc fragments pressing on the nerve roots. This exploration is usually done at more than one level to ensure that the spinal nerve roots going to the legs are completely free of any entrapment.

is extremely risky; sometimes the surgery must be performed through the chest or the abdomen to approach the vertebra from in front. Malignant tumors usually threaten a patient's life; however, if they are discovered early, a cure is occasionally possible or the quality of the patient's life can at least be very much improved.

Surgery for Trauma With the advent of high-speed vehicles, especially motorcycles, more and more patients are sustaining spinal injuries. People who are thrown from a vehicle after a sudden deceleration-type accident are almost always severely injured. Serious head and spine injuries are often sustained. These injuries can be avoided by using a seat belt that has both a lap and shoulder restraint. Get yourself into the habit of buckling up your seat belt *every time* you get into your car! Studies have shown that 80 percent of all serious automobile injuries occur within a twenty-five-mile radius of the home.

Fractures of the spine in the neck can occur as a result of sudden flexion and extension. The cervical vertebrae are crushed or dislocated (a fracture dislocation). If the injury is mild, the patient will develop palsy or weakness and pain in either the upper or lower extremities, or in both. If the injury is severe enough and occurs high in the neck, the patient will rarely survive. Severe injury lower in the neck—in the region of the fifth, sixth, or seventh cervical vertebrae—causes paralysis in both the upper and lower extremities and loss of bladder and bowel control.

Fracture dislocations lower in the spine usually occur in the lower thoracic or upper lumbar region. If the injury is mild, the spinal cord and nerve roots will not be affected. Spinal fusion should be promptly done if the fracture is unstable. Usually metal rods, springs, or wires are used to weld the fractured vertebrae together. Occasionally a synthetic cement that sets at an extremely rapid rate is used to provide additional stability. Generally the two vertebrae above and two below the unstable area are included in the fusion. When the spinal cord itself is injured, fusion is indicated to prevent further injury to the cord and to facilitate nursing tasks such as helping the patient out of bed and into a wheelchair.

Occasionally reports of surgery to hook up a severed spinal cord surface. These reports are totally false; it is virtually impossible to splice a severed spinal cord together again. Exploratory surgery in a patient who is paralyzed as a result of a spinal cord injury is almost always a worthless surgical endeavor. The only time it is warranted is when some nerve function remains and CT scanning and myelography indicate that direct bony pressure is increasing the damage to the cord. Surgical decompression can then help reverse neurologic damage and improve the patient's condition. In almost all instances, spinal fusion is done at the same time or two weeks later.

In most cases of spinal injury both a neurosurgeon and an orthopaedic surgeon work as a team to effect a proper treatment for the patient. If the patient has been paralyzed, a long rehabilitation period—including months in the hospital to learn to walk with braces and crutches—will be necessary before the patient is able to resume a reasonably normal life.

Surgery for Infections Occasionally patients have an infection that was carried through the bloodstream to the spine. For instance, a severe throat or kidney infection can spread to the spine, usually to the body of the vertebra, where it causes disability and pain.

Today, tuberculosis of the spine is uncommon and can usually be adequately treated with antibiotics. Spinal fusion is rarely required. However, decompression may be necessary for other infectious diseases if the spinal cord or nerves are entrapped. The decompression can be made either through a needle-type probe such as an arthroscope or through direct visualization during an open operation. If the causative bacterium is identified, the patient is placed on appropriate antibiotics and in most instances completely cured. Occasionally infections become chronic and require extensive surgery with antibiotic therapy to prevent osteomyelitis, a chronic bone infection.

On rare occasions a wound infection develops after surgery. The wound must then be adequately drained and antibiotics given. Usually the wound must be flushed with antibiotic solutions, a suction-irrigation technique. With treatment, patients usually do quite well.

Anterior Spinal Surgery

All the operations discussed thus far are done from the back (the posterior approach). However, there are instances where surgery must be done from the front of the spine (the anterior approach). An anterior approach is indicated in congenital problems when there is so little bone left in the posterior part of the spine that it is impossible to do an adequate decompression or spinal fusion from the back. Other indications for the anterior approach are chronic posterior infections where further posterior surgery would be unsafe, and conditions where the spinal cord or nerve roots are compressed by either a tumor or tuberculous infection and an anterior decompression is essential.

For the anterior procedure, the spine is approached through the rib cage or the abdomen. Most often a rib is removed and used later on as a bone graft to stabilize the spine from in front. In the lumbar spine, the incision is through the abdomen, either along the midline or along one side near the kidney. The lower spine can be effectively decompressed and stabilized through this incision. In general, anterior spinal surgery is slightly more hazardous and complicated than posterior surgery. An anterior approach should only be used when absolutely necessary.

WHAT TO EXPECT FROM SURGERY—PROGNOSIS

The success of spinal surgery depends on many factors. First of all, the skill of the technician performing your surgery is of prime importance. An exerienced surgeon will obtain a better result than an inexperienced one. Secondly, it is important that the right operation be done for proper indications. Ideally, a single operation should be all that is required. During this one operation, all necessary constructive and corrective procedures should be done. An ill-conceived, ill-designed procedure that is improperly executed by a poor technician will almost always need to be repeated.

It is important not to expect too much from surgery. If goals are unrealistic, the surgery will be a failure for psychological reasons. If a person has been having chronic, disabling back pain for the past ten or fifteen years, it is unrealistic to expect complete relief of pain after surgery. It is best if both you and your surgeon agree on goals prior to surgery.

In most cases where surgery is done by a skilled technician for specific pathology, the results will be excellent. The patient's back pain will decrease and he will have a permanently stable and relatively pain-free back for the rest of his life. Surgery does not rejuvenate, however. Do not expect your back to be able to withstand unusual stresses and strains for the next twenty years without giving you some symptoms. Back pain may also recur as a result of another problem elsewhere in the spine.

LIFE AFTER SPINAL SURGERY

Sexual Activity

Most people are concerned about sexual activity during an episode of back pain and after spinal surgery. In general, with a little bit of ingenuity, sexual activity does not have to be curtailed at all, even during an episode of acute backache. As I have mentioned in the exercise section of this book, the pelvic tilt (the first PRE) is one of the exercises that relieves most back pain. This exercise resembles the gentle pelvic motions of sexual activity. I am not recommending that a person with back pain be overly active during sexual activity, but certainly he or she can assume a passive role. Both partners can lie on their sides with the man approaching from in back. This is called the *spoon position*; it can be used without aggravating existing back pain. Naturally, when a person has suffered an acute spinal injury and is in extreme muscle pain, a sympathetic mate won't insist on unreasonable gratification until the partner is more comfortable.

Sexual activity can usually be resumed within the first two weeks after spinal surgery. Again, the side or spoon position is usually most comfortable and least demanding. A firm mattress is important so that the spine does not sag excessively. A small pillow under the small of the back or under the waist can also be helpful. Sexual relations can begin as early as ten or twelve days after surgery if the couple goes about it gently and avoids any activity that might cause an increase in pain.

Diet Control

After spinal surgery, diet is most important. Fortunately, most people lose weight at the time of surgery and leave the hospital five to ten pounds lighter than when they arrived. In most cases, patients should work to keep this weight off. The majority of patients I see are overweight and underexercised. They should be pleased to have a head start on their weight-control program and strive to regain strength without regaining weight. A proper diet supplemented with adequate mineral and vitamin supplements will satisfy the body's needs without adding excess weight.

Most patients lose blood during their operation, and it is therefore essential that they take multivitamins with iron so that the blood cells can rapidly re-form within three or four weeks. Generally a multivitamin with iron in the morning and evening for a three-month period should satisfy these needs.

A Cautionary Approach to Life

Once you have undergone spinal surgery, you are sure to want to avoid going through it again. With reasonable sense, your spinal operation should last you the rest of your life. If you have been fortunate enough to have a good early postoperative result, you should protect that result by living cautiously, especially when it comes to physical activities. Most people try to do too much, too soon. Avoid the temptation to overdo or you may reinjure your back and require further surgery in the future. It takes approximately six months for a spinal fusion to become solid. Most fusions start getting solid between the third to fifth month. A serious fall or stressful physical activity during this period could endanger the success of the operation.

After spinal surgery, remember to squat to pick things up—never bend forward. If you have groceries in the trunk of your car, never bend over the trunk to lift them. This puts undue stresses on the spine. Don't do stupid things like lifting a heavy lawn mower into the back of the car or strenuous yard chores that involve prolonged bending, digging, or swinging an ax. Always keep in mind the major insult your body has sustained. Your fusion will not become solid unless you take good care of it. Eat properly and take recommended mineral supplements. At the same time, slowly increase the stresses you put on your spine. Avoid sudden movement and situations for which you are physically unprepared.

Reduced Emotional Stress

It is also important that you keep emotional stresses to a minimum. It is unrealistic to expect stress to go away, but you can modify stresses and try to cope with them better so that they will be less harmful to you psychologically and physically.

Adjust Your Job to Your Back or Your Back to Your Job

If you have a difficult job that involves prolonged standing or bending, it has probably contributed to your back problem. If this is the case, you should try to find some other job that will not harm your weak back, or you will jeopardize the success of your recent spinal surgery. Obviously, you should avoid heavy labor for fear of reinjuring your back. If it is impossible for you to get lighter work, you will have to quit that job and find another more suitable one. If you have chronic back problems, you do not want a job where you have to be constantly on your feet or where there is prolonged bending and stooping. If you have been a productive employee, most employers are more than happy to adjust your job to your spinal condition.

Exercise

You can begin a regular exercise program once your spinal fusion has healed. The five KPEs (Keim Preventive Exercises) and six PREs (Pain-Relieving Exercises) will be most helpful and can be started six months after your operation. Doing these exercises gently, on a daily basis, will help strengthen your spinal muscles and improve your physical well-being tremendously. You will have spent two weeks in the hospital and another six months nursing your back to proper spinal health. Your spinal muscles will be weak and exercises will be most important. Be sure to do your exercises every day for the rest of your life.

THE MULTIPLY OPERATED BACK—WHY?

Each week I see three or four patients in my office who already have had a minimum of three or four back operations. Why does this happen? Obviously, the very first operation is the most important one. If the wrong operation was done for the wrong indications originally, the most skilled technician will fail in his attempt to improve the situation. If the right operation was done for the right indications but the technician was poorly qualified, the operation will probably be a failure. Sometimes the situation the surgeon tried to correct is really not correctable. Even the most skilled surgeon cannot correct certain physical conditions. Sometimes patients have psychological problems that have prompted surgery that should not have been done in the first place. These people keep returning for more and more surgery. Some actually are masochistic and thrive on repeated pain.

Most commonly, the multiply operated patient has had a poor result from his first operation. A second attempt was made that for various reasons also failed. A third, fourth, and even fifth procedure sometimes follows. By that time, adhesions have formed and the patient has memorized pain patterns so deeply in the psyche that it is absolutely impossible to dislodge them. In these instances, even the finest surgery, carried out by the most skilled technician for the best indications, will still result in failure. Many of these patients have already become narcotic addicts or alcoholics. In these cases no further attempts at surgery should be made and the patient should be referred to a pain clinic.

PAIN CLINICS

In the United States there are many clinics that treat patients with chronic pain. Pain treatment centers try to evaluate the patient's entire being. They make a psychological assessment and review all spinal problems, using X rays, CT scans, and myelograms. Often further neurological tests are performed to see if there is any real physical (organic) problem that has been overlooked and is treatable. Unfortunately, further surgery is almost never an option for the multiply operated patient. Pain clinics try to find out if there is any secondary gain or psychological motivation present in the patient's pain syndrome. Most patients are given psychiatric testing in an effort to detect the underlying reasons for chronic pain.

Some pain clinics treat people as inpatients for a period of two to four weeks. All medications are given to the professional personnel of the clinic. They then meter out the medications in ever-decreasing doses so that the patient is ultimately weaned from intoxicating and addictive drugs. This is one of the most important functions of the pain control clinics and can be done most effectively. Clinics may offer consultations with psychiatrists and neurologists to help you cope with your pain.

Simply put, these pain programs offer a new way of life. The patient is expected to adhere to the treatments and principles of pain clinics once he has returned home. The adjustment can be difficult for the patient and his family. However, people with a sincere desire to lead a pain-free life must follow, to the letter, the recommendations given.

Pain clinics are located at the University of Virginia Medical Center in Charlottesville, Virginia; the Johns Hopkins University School of Medicine Pain Clinic in Baltimore, Maryland; the Pain Clinic at the University of Illinois College of Medicine in Chicago, Illinois; the Pain Clinic at the Rush Medical College at the Rush-Presbyterian-St. Luke's Medical Center in Chicago; the Pain Center at the City of Hope National Medical Center in Duarte, California; the Pain Consultation Clinic of the Mt. Sinai Medical Center in Miami Beach, Florida; the Pain Management Center of Mayo Clinic in Rochester, Minnesota; the Pain and Health Rehabilitation Center in La-Crosse, Wisconsin; the Pain Clinic at the University of Washington School of Medicine in Seattle, Washington; the Pain Treatment Clinic at UCLA School of Medicine in Los Angeles; the Pain Clinic at the Mt. Zion Hospital and Medical Center in San Francisco, California; the Pain Clinic Center of the Mesa-Lutheran Hospital in Mesa, Arizona; the Pain Unit of the Massachusetts Rehabilitation Hospital in Boston; the Portland Pain Rehabilitation Center of the Emmanuel Hospital in Portland, Oregon; the Pain Clinic of the Georgetown Medical Center in Washington, D.C.; the Pain Clinic at the Columbia-Presbyterian Medical Center in New York City; and finally, the Nebraska Pain Rehabilitation Unit at the University of Nebraska in Omaha.

More pain clinics are springing up every year and are usually staffed by extremely conscientious and highly professional people. You will not only find there the warmth and understanding that is necessary for your rehabilitation, but people who are professionals and most competent.

If you have had chronic disabling pain and you have had spinal surgery which has failed for various reasons, the combination of treatments given at these pain centers can, if closely adhered to, change your way of life and turn a disastrous result into a satisfactory one.

Ten

HOW TO CARE FOR YOUR BACK— SUMMARY

The past chapters have described the causes of backache and their management. Although great medical advances have occurred in the past eighty years, the future looks even brighter.

A great deal of medical research is being done regarding pain mechanisms. We know how *subjective* pain is and that some people experience more or less pain than others. Researchers must find out what makes one person more pain-free and stoical than his neighbor. Chemicals such as beta-endorphin must be more carefully investigated to see if more effective and safer pain-relieving drugs cannot be found.

Pain clinics will eventually tally enough information from computer studies to elucidate pain patterns, how to avoid them, and how to cope with them. Behavior modification will be available to help us become more aware of pain cycles—what sets them off and how to stop them before they start.

A greater awareness of stress in the home and on the job, with better-established coping mechanisms, will certainly be a great future aid. Employers are more aware of the mental and physical needs of their employees. They now stress emotional balance and satisfaction as well as physical fitness programs. Some even offer financial benefits to employees who break the cigarette habit or lose substantial weight.

Research into more sophisticated medical techniques, both nonoperative and surgical, will be constantly forthcoming. Better medical care ensures aggressive preventive medicine and is evident from better designs in furniture for office and home as well as orthopaedic auto and airplane seats. Medical research is always looking for easier ways to prevent medical problems before they start or to minimize them once they occur. The future is bright, but the problem is complicated and difficult.

CONCLUSIONS

By this time, you should have an adequate knowledge of what your back is all about and how to relieve back pain if you have it. If you are fortunate enough not to have suffered back pain, I hope you will start the five Keim Preventive Exercises (KPEs) so you can *prevent* back trouble. If you are already a victim of back pain, you should start the six Pain-Relieving Exercises (PREs). These will help you get through acute or chronic bouts of back pain. As mentioned before, the five KPEs and six PREs can be easily performed in about twenty minutes and *if done daily* should keep you out of the doctor's office. That is the main aim of my book!

The three major culprits producing backache are stress, improper diet, and lack of proper exercise. You should now realize that you can alter these factors and thus reduce your chance of getting back pain. If you adhere to the suggestions I have laid down for you, by now you should be adequately informed as to what you can do to help yourself. If your self-diagnosis and treatment fail you, the section describing how to choose the proper doctor to help you manage your problem should fill your need.

In most cases, you will be able to achieve a healthy back either through self-help or with a doctor's intervention. It is rare that you will need to resort to surgery for a spinal problem; I estimate that only 1 or 2 percent of all patients with back problems actually require surgery. In many instances people who require surgery, if given enough time for nature to run through the normal healing process, will actually be able to defer or avoid surgery completely.

"Lifetime spinal care" is the theme of this book. By now you should understand how important it is to keep the muscles of your spine properly nourished and exercised. People who will spend a minimum period of fifteen minutes a day doing the

KPEs, eat proper foods, and try to cope with emotional stress will enjoy a life free of back pain.

A lifetime of proper spinal care will become increasingly important as the general population grows. Most women now live into the mideighties; most men survive into the late seventies or early eighties. If our bodies are to withstand the ravages of aging and abuse, we will have to maintain them as perfectly as possible. We get only one spine to last us for an entire life. Taking proper care of your spine should be your lifetime goal, and reducing the abuses that naturally occur should be something that is paramount in your mind.

If spinal problems affect you or members of your family, you can refer to this book to help you solve them. By adjusting your life and following the exercise and health program, you should be able to realize a lifetime of good spinal health.

Index

Numbers of pages on which illustrations occur are in *italics*.